self-care

for the

real world

for Mum and Dad

self-care

for the

real world

nadia narain
&
katia narain phillips

abrams image, new york

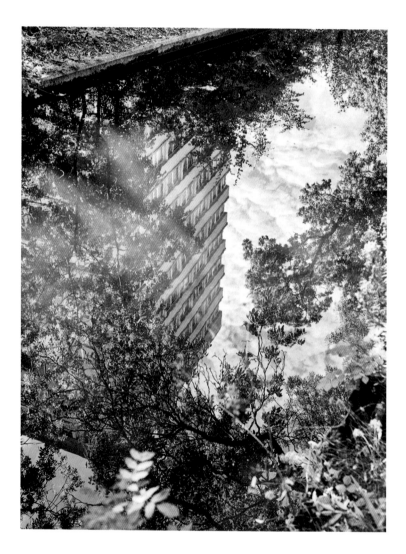

CONTENTS

WHAT IS SELF-CARE?

'I have come to believe that caring for myself is not self-indulgent, caring for myself is an act of survival.' Audre Lorde

At the most basic level, self-care means the ability to get yourself fed, dressed and washed, and to generally function in the world. Everyone practises self-care, even if they're not aware of it. In this book, we want to help you learn how to turn self-care into something that is not just about functioning but flourishing. The way we like to define self-care is learning to look after your own self as you would a child or a very dear friend – with love, kindness and patience.

We use the word caring as a compliment, yet when we talk about self-care, sometimes people assume it means only caring for oneself, regardless of the impact on others. We have even heard people say that self-care is selfish. But we believe if you feel you are the best version of yourself, you will have more to give and to contribute to the world. When we feel good about ourselves we do better, kinder things for ourselves and for others, and we naturally let the good things in our lives grow. When we feel bad, we become more selfish and self-absorbed and we don't have the energy to give to other people or to the things or causes we care about.

Self-care can sometimes seem like it's just a hashtag for wellness influencers on Instagram, but we want you to remember that self-care isn't just for people who have hours of spare time, or lots of money for expensive massages or pedicures. You don't have to put off self-care until your life is less busy, or until you've perfected your diet, or bought those fancy yoga leggings.

To us, self-care means being switched on, fully present and engaged in your life. It's the opposite of switching off and retreating from the world. Ignoring your own needs leaves you depleted, but self-care will energise and recharge you.

This is the real world, and there will always be demands on your time and energy. But you are deserving of a little of your time and energy, just as much as anyone else around you. Self-care doesn't mean overhauling your entire life in a drastic way – who has time for that? It's about meeting yourself where you are right now, instead of where you think you should be, and thinking about the small steps you can take to care for yourself better. You might be surprised at how transformative just a few small steps can be.

So remember, self-care is not selfish. It is all about learning self-love, self-respect, self-compassion and seeing the impact that all of these have on your own wellbeing, and the wellbeing of those around you.

This book is full of the ideas that have worked for us over the years and we hope they'll inspire you, too.

WHAT IS SELF-CARE TO YOU?

You probably already know the basics: move your body, feed your body, nourish your mind and soul. But it's important to remember that self-care is going to feel different for everyone.

The best way to nail what self-care means to you is learning to know the difference between what you need rather than what you want. Getting what you want can feel superficial – whether it's the latest iPhone or a great pair of shoes. It may give you an instant buzz but it won't sustain you long term. Getting what you need goes a little deeper.

Words like nourish, nurture, resource, recharge, refuel, love and kindness are the essence of self-care. Remind yourself of these words when you're reaching towards a want – stop and ask yourself, is this nurturing me? Is this refuelling me? Is this recharging me?

Look for the balance; it's important to check in with everything that's going on with your life so you can get a holistic view and tweak things accordingly.

Self-care will mean different things to you at different times in your life. If something big is going on – a break-up, a bereavement, a house move – you will need to take care of yourself in a kind and gentle way; if things are going well and you have some spare time and energy, the best self-care might be to challenge yourself a little.

Remember, no one else's way is the right way for you. Not even our way! Which is why this book is about helping you find what works for you.

TAKING CARE OF YOURSELF
IS NOT OPTIONAL

Our mission is not about achieving perfection, it's about accepting you are human, with all your beauty and all your flaws, accepting you deserve to be happy and well, and doing what you can, when you can, to get there.

We know from experience that magical thinking doesn't work, and neither does blindly trying to be positive – sometimes chanting positive affirmations when you're feeling terrible can even make you feel worse. What is most effective is learning what works for you, and identifying the small, powerful changes you can make which will transform the way you feel.

Learning to feel good can feel weird if you're not used to it. Maybe you have somehow learned to believe that you don't deserve to be looked after. But you do – and you are the first and best person to do it.

You know what they tell you about the oxygen mask in the safety demonstration on a plane? That you have to put on yours before you put on your child's? We didn't understand that for years, but the more we learnt about self-care, the more we got it that if the parent didn't put on their mask first in an emergency, their child wouldn't survive. This is true for all kinds of things in life; if you are depleted and exhausted emotionally, physically or mentally you will have nothing to give anyone else.

Think of it as survival of the most resilient: right now you may be deep in the waves of life, being tossed around. Learning self-care is like building your own lifeboat, plank by plank; once you've got your boat, you'll still be rocked by the same waves but you'll have a feeling of safety, and a stability that means you can pick up other people on your way.

LEARN WHAT YOU NEED

The first step of self-care is to pay attention. Start to listen to what your body needs, and how it reacts, and you will begin to hone your intuition. Through the course of this book the exercises we suggest will get you closer to reading and understanding your body.

It's not easy, we know, when you're being bombarded with information about what you should be doing, or what you should or shouldn't eat. Do you have a tendency to try something that's popular – like giving up sugar, perhaps – then insist on everyone else trying it too? We used to do that. But there is no one prescription and different things work for different people at different times. If you just do the things that other people tell you to, they may not give you the energy or relaxation you crave. Or the results won't last, if your new habits are not truly in line with what you need.

You may be so busy that you haven't checked in with yourself for a while. Do you really want to do a spin class after work, or are you going because you think you should? Is a fourth coffee or tea today a habit or a necessity? (If you say it's a necessity, we'll work on getting you properly rested in a later chapter!) Why are you eating that family-sized bar of chocolate – for pleasure? Or did you get into a fight with someone and now there's a big empty feeling inside that you're trying to fill?

We are going to teach you to read your body, so that at every point you can check in to find out what is going to work. Trust us, your body knows.

OUR OWN SELF-CARE

Our own paths to self-care have been long, with plenty of detours, and we have learned lessons the hard way. Having practised yoga, reiki and massage from a young age, we got really good at looking after other people way before we learned to look after ourselves!

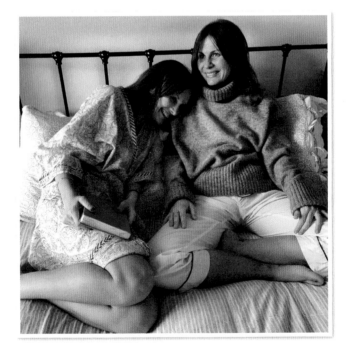

WE LOVE LISTS!

In Matt Haig's book *Reasons to Stay Alive*, he explains how he created lists to help with his anxiety and depression. He wrote a list of things that made him feel bad, and a list of things that made him feel better. As soon as we read these, we started making our own self-care lists, writing down the things that make us feel terrible, and those that make us feel good and grounded. We've combined our lists because we are both pretty similar – apart from cooking (Katia's thing) and meditating (only Nadia likes it).

What's on your list? Write it down.

OUR NON-SELF-CARE LIST

* Too many late nights in a row.
* Thinking we should be somewhere other than where we are.
* Pretending to be anything other than ourselves.
* Comparing ourselves to other people.
* Not paying attention to our bodies.
* Eating too much sugar.
* Eating junk food.
* Working too much.
* Not practising yoga enough.
* Forgetting to meditate because I've been on Instagram for too long.
* Zoning out to box sets.
* TV in general.
* Social media in general.
* Not taking a day off when we need to.
* Missing meals.
* Not being around friends and family.
* Being around too many people for too long.

OUR SELF-CARE LIST

* Making sure we get to bed by 10.30 most nights.
* Taking a relaxing bath or shower before bed.
* Preparing ahead when it comes to food so that we eat healthy and tasty things.
* Being around friends and family.
* Dancing.
* Going to yoga class.
* Meditating every day (Nadia).
* Doing our gratitude journals every morning and night.
* Being honest to ourselves about ourselves.
* Paying attention to self-critical thoughts and changing the track to something more positive.
* Treating ourselves as kindly as we treat the people we teach and feed.
* Taking naps and rest when needed.
* Walking in nature.
* Swimming in the sea.
* Having quiet time.

love

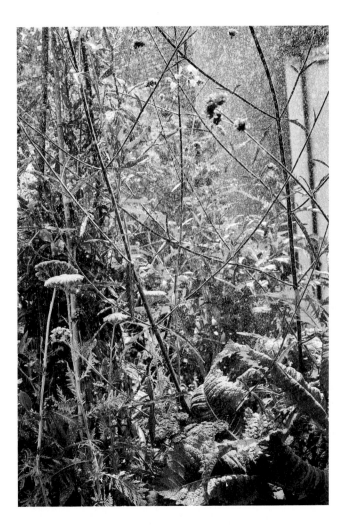

'Just for a while, be open to the possibility that there is nothing wrong with you.' *Cheri Huber*

You might think loving yourself sounds a bit self-indulgent, but when you practise it fully it puts more responsibility for your life on you and so relieves the pressure on the people you love. Self-love is not narcissism or self-centredness, it is a kindness to yourself and also to those around you. It means you won't go around looking for love in other people or things, or hoping that others will fill the emptiness you think you have inside.

We can make the mistake of thinking that love only means romantic love, and that if we don't have that great romance in our life right now, it must mean we're unloved and unlovable. This is why self-love, and self-care in love, are a big deal; they're the type of love you can always be sure will be there for you, no matter what.

Putting care and love into yourself will allow you to be more open to receiving love from others, and you will find you have more to give. It's like a circle, and it starts with you.

Some lucky people learnt to love themselves in childhood, but the rest of us have to learn it along the way, at different stages of our life. We hope this section will help you.

THERE IS NOTHING WRONG WITH YOU

'What if I forgave myself? What if I forgave myself even though I'd done some things I shouldn't have? What if all those things I shouldn't have done were what got me here? What if I was never redeemed? What if I already was?' *Cheryl Strayed*

Just imagine, for a minute, that this statement is completely true: there is nothing wrong with you. Say it a few times. See how it feels. Weird, right?

A lot of us are brought up to believe we need to be better in some way. Maybe you were told that you should get top grades at school, or maybe there was something you felt you had to achieve in order to please someone you loved. That's fine if you got the message you were still lovable, even if you failed the exam or got suspended from school, but if the overall message you heard from your parents or significant people around you was that love had conditions attached, it may be hard, even as an adult, to ever feel you're good enough.

Don't get us wrong, we do believe in working hard and doing your best, but what also matters is not so much that you can *be* good, more that you were *already* born full of goodness and love.

Other things that have happened to you may lead you to think there's something wrong with you. A boyfriend may have said one small thing about you when you were going out, and it stuck. Even if you haven't seen him for years, you may still feel that part of you needs to be fixed or changed. Nadia remembers her best friend in school telling her she should always wear baggy clothes and cover up her legs because they were too skinny. It was only when, as an adult, a friend asked why she always hid her body that she remembered it, and realised it had stayed with her for years.

So think about what early messages you absorbed about yourself. Can you begin to question those messages and ask if they are really true?

Those childhood patterns stay with us, and when we are reminded of them by something that happens in the present, we often find ourselves coming back to the same ingrained message: there is something wrong with me. When something happens in adult life to confirm this – maybe criticism from a boss, or a row with a partner or a friend – we find ourselves dragged into the painful place in our minds where we feel we are not good enough.

Remember that even if you've behaved badly, or have done something mean or unkind, that does not make you a terrible person. We all make mistakes. The most self-caring thing you can do right now is forgive yourself.

HOW TO MAKE FRIENDS WITH YOUR THOUGHTS

You may have tried all kinds of ways to escape this feeling of not being good enough. People look for a magic wand to make the pain or empty feeling go away. Maybe you go shopping to feel better, or drink a lot, or have sex with people you don't like much (because you want them to like you). Or perhaps you go to a tarot card reader in the hope of hearing that things will change because of fate or destiny, rather than because of your own actions.

Some people keep going to different therapists, buying self-help books, going on retreats, visiting gurus and healers, going on diets or fasts, or searching for a way to feel okay about themselves. We understand this – we did this too! And none of this is wrong in itself, but it's hard to hear the voice inside if you're always looking for your answers outside.

You will never be rid of the stuff you don't like, but what if you learn that your flaws are beautiful and you can be friends with them?

That's not to say there's anything wrong with wanting to change some behavioural patterns that don't work for you. Nor that you shouldn't learn new ways to be and to grow. What we're saying is, there's a difference between practising self-care because you think you're a shitty person who needs fixing, and practising self-care because you are treating yourself in the same way you would treat someone you love.

Think about why you are doing yoga or meditating or exercising, or changing your diet. Be honest. Are you trying to fix something? Or can you learn to see that you're perfect as you are, with all your flaws and your beauty? Don't practise self-care to fix yourself, do it out of great love and respect for the person you are and the body you live in.

WHAT DO YOU LIKE
ABOUT YOURSELF?

Write a list of three to five things you like about yourself. If you get stuck, think of someone you love and write three to five things about them instead. See how easy that is? Now, think about you again . . .

The first few times you do this it may feel tricky, but it will get easier.

To start you off, here is an example:

* I care about other people.

* I like to make people laugh.

* I am loyal.

Now do your own list and see how it feels.

Once you've done this, write down three to five things you have done that make you feel proud of yourself.

HOW TO MANAGE THE BLACK HOLE

There will always be some things that trigger you emotionally. It's human nature to experience pain and loneliness and fear. They are a part of you. The feeling that you are not enough may always come up, but there is a way to deal with it that will leave you feeling like you *are* enough.

The distinction you want to make is this: it could be you've done something wrong, or something has gone wrong, but there is nothing wrong with you.

Here's how the process works:

* Notice when you feel a negative emotion. This may seem strange at first, because you'll be sitting outside your thoughts, looking in on your life. Human beings have what's called negative bias, where we ignore the good stuff and focus on the bad. If you don't notice your negative bias, and your reaction to it, your not-good-enough button gets pressed.

* So next time you feel an emotional reaction to something someone's said or done, first notice it. State it to yourself as clearly as this: 'Oh, here we go.' Watch yourself react.

* Then notice this: how long does it take from the moment when that feeling is triggered to when it starts to dissipate? An hour, a day, a week? Notice when you try to distract yourself from your dark feeling in your usual way: maybe by shopping, eating or being bad-tempered with someone you love.

* Instead, sit with the feeling. It will suck, it will feel awful, but watch it, as if you were watching a crap movie. Then notice as it changes . . . and realise it won't last.

This does take a load of practice and effort, and you may not be able to do it first time. We both have to practise this constantly, having businesses that get publicly reviewed and commented on. We had to learn how to focus on the good stuff and to take the negatives as constructive criticism, showing us how we could improve.

And, if it's really hard, why not ask someone you love to give you some much-needed perspective?

LEARNING TO LIVE WITH THE PARTS YOU DON'T LIKE

Think about the qualities you don't like in yourself. Your anxiety? Loneliness? Paranoia? It's going to feel strange, but those are the things you need to make friends with. Perfection isn't what makes people attractive, it's your flaws and vulnerability that make you, you.

> Katia: 'I'm prone to imposter syndrome. When I start preparing a dinner party for a client, or if I'm creating new recipes for the café, I find myself thinking, this is it: this time everyone will find out that I can't actually cook. It feels very real. The pressure brings out my insecurity and then I think I'm an imposter. I started to feel better about it when I read that it's very common with successful women. That means I might be successful, right?!'

> Nadia: 'I used to get super sad when bad things happened and I'd be afraid I couldn't shift it. But once I accepted that sadness is part of my make-up and I worked on how to look after myself during those bouts, it became more manageable.

> 'Now when that feeling comes I think, "Oh shit, here it is". And I get things in place to make it feel softer, not unlike you would if you were dealing with a child who was sad. You would make sure they felt loved and looked after, that they had nice things to do, and someone to talk to.'

WHAT HAPPENS WHEN YOU TRULY BELIEVE THERE IS NOTHING WRONG WITH YOU?

Something quite wonderful. You like who you are more, and it shows. People notice it. You feel comfortable in your skin and in your being, and that is a very attractive quality. Being vulnerable is not a weakness. We all have stuff we don't like about ourselves, and when we are able to be open and honest about our vulnerabilities, we realise we are not alone in our feelings. Repeat after me: there is nothing wrong with me.

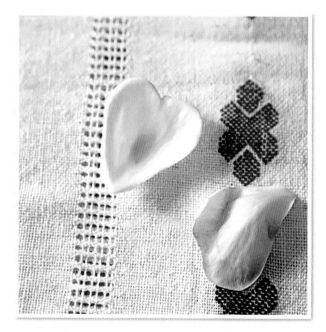

IT'S TIME TO LOVE YOUR BODY

'I can't overestimate the importance of accepting ourselves exactly as we are right now, not as we wish we were or think we ought to be.' Pema Chodron

We're not expecting you to fall in love with your body overnight. What we'd like you to do first is notice what you think about yourself when you look in the mirror. Most of us immediately clock something we don't like: urgh, my ass is too big, I look old, my nose is wrong, why the fuck is one eye smaller than the other? This is the loop that plays in most people's minds, and we're yet to meet someone who doesn't play a version of that old tune.

Being stuck in this groove is not self-care. It is, as you well know, actually being really, really mean to yourself. Would you stand in front of the mirror with your best friend and look at her and say all the things to her that you are saying about yourself? No bloody way! She would be in tears and never want to talk to you again. So why do you think it's okay to be like that about yourself? You're sending yourself a negative message every time you catch your reflection in a shop window, or the car mirror.

So, stand in front of a mirror and try to change the script. It will feel strange at first, but keep going. With practice you'll start to be kinder to your body and less critical of yourself.

* Do you see that there is no one now, or ever will be, anyone on this planet quite like you?

* Can you look at your eyes and thank them for all the beauty they see for you?

* What about your incredible nose, so clever with the aromas it smells and the breath it takes that can send signals to your brain and change your mood?

* That mouth! All that it gets to say, to taste, to inspire.

* All the lines on your face, the lived-in memories of your time on this planet.

* Oh, and then there is that insane body of yours. Its own unique shape. It can give you such incredible pleasure. It heals itself when it is hurt. It breathes for you all day and night without you ever having to remember to turn your breath on or off. It allows you to swim in oceans and climb mountains, to make love and share joy. Think of what it does for you daily, even when you don't take care of it, even when you criticize it or wish it looked like someone else's body.

* Look at your reflection. Can you be kind rather than critical?

PAY ATTENTION!

Have you ever noticed how babies have a different cry for each of the things they need? One cry might mean she wants milk, one that she's tired, another that she's uncomfortable, and if you ignore the cries, they get louder and louder, more and more distraught. If you've spent time with a baby, you might have, through trial and error, finally learnt what each cry means. But can you identify your own cries or signs? And do you take notice of them?

By the time you're an adult you've got a whole load of different cries – for hunger, thirst or tiredness, but also on an emotional level. For example, you might need love or comfort or reassurance. There are a whole lot of buttons that can get pressed by life, but can you tell your cries apart, or do you let your needs play out, or do you just ignore them?

We have to be so controlled as adult human beings. Remember the last time you felt like crying? If you were in the office or anywhere public you probably had to keep it together. You couldn't, like a toddler, wail and hold out your arms and expect to be picked up and comforted.

Do you notice what you feel like if you miss a meal? Do you get short-tempered, grumpy or hangry? What happens if you don't drink enough water; do you feel tired and sluggish? If you drink too much coffee or tea, do you feel jittery and a bit agitated?

The way to understand your body's cries is by checking in with yourself regularly and working out what you need . . . before things get to tantrum stage.

HOW TO CHECK IN WITH YOUR BODY

Try doing this body scan a few times today. It's so powerful; it gives you very clear information but it doesn't need to take more than 30 seconds. You may want to make it a regular habit.

This is all you do:

Sit still with your feet on the ground, eyes closed. Notice your body and pay attention to your breath. How do you feel? How is your energy? What is your posture like? Are you clenching your jaw? Or any other part of your body? What is your mood? Do you have any pain, discomfort or tension? How do you feel emotionally? Are you craving sugar or tea or coffee? Don't judge, just notice.

When you've truly noticed how you feel, ask yourself how you could feel better. Do you need to drink more water? Do you need to step away from the computer and walk around for a couple of minutes?

If you feel pain, that is a warning signal from your body. Don't ignore it. Go to the doctor, or to a physiotherapist or osteopath. Pain is your body shouting for attention. Paying attention before you get to this point can save you from making things worse.

Scanning helps you to take notice. Only then can you figure out what to do to feel better. A lot of self-care is about noticing, and you'll find this gets super simple with practice.

DO SOMETHING FOR YOUR
BODY AND MIND

We are firm believers that how you look is a reflection of how you feel. When you feel good about yourself, you look amazing. When you don't feel good about yourself, nothing looks good.

Next time you do something to care for your body, whether it's exercise or rest, a massage or a nice long bath, notice how you feel afterwards. Are you feeling kinder towards yourself? Do you look at yourself with different eyes? Are you more likely to see the good things?

It's strange but true: you may not look any different, the dark circles or wrinkles or whatever your mind used to fixate on will likely still be there, but you will see yourself differently. Your lens will have softened; your new focus has given you a new perspective.

That's the power of self-care: do it and you will experience the incredible feedback loop that changes your thoughts, too . . . which in turn makes you want to look after yourself more.

How we feel about our looks is filtered through how we feel, full stop. When we feel good, we like ourselves. Keep doing the stuff that makes you feel good.

MASSAGE - A NECESSITY,
NOT A LUXURY

People think of massage as a luxury – so self-indulgent, a waste of money. But massage, even self-massage, is an amazing tool for helping you to have a better relationship with your body.

We think it's the best birthday present you could possibly give or have – to show your body some love. It can feel like a lot of money to spend, especially when you don't have something to show for it, like a new pair of shoes, but think of a massage as an investment in your health and wellbeing.

If you can't afford to pay for a massage, you could ask a friend or your partner to swap massages with you. You don't have to be a professional therapist to give someone a good shoulder rub. Maybe your child, or your friend, could massage your feet?

Or you could do this soothing stomach massage on yourself. We learned it from Tanya Goodman, who calls it the Belly Love Method. It's very calming, as well as being great therapy for an irritable bowel or an upset stomach. You can do this massage while clothed or not, it's up to you.

Warm up: Seated or standing, begin by vigorously rubbing your palms together until they feel warm. Then make your hands into fists and rub up and down the front of the thighs seven times or so with your knuckles.

Tune in: Place your right palm flat beneath your right rib; this is the area of your liver. Place your left palm on top of your right. Your thumbs should be near your lowest right rib, one on top of the other. This is position one.

Take a slow, deep breath and tune into the rise and fall of your hands. Encourage the breath to rise up from the little fingers to the thumbs. Connect to the shapes and sensations beneath your hands. Encourage your whole belly to rise on the inhale and come back down on the exhale.

Avoid forcing your belly out with your muscles. Imagine instead that you are breathing from your lower belly all the way to your chest: a nice big breath.

Circles: Picture your abdomen with two circles drawn on it: one above the belly button to just below the ribs, and one below your belly button to the bottom of your abdomen.

For the upper belly: With your palms in position one on the right rib, thumbs touching – circle your hands clockwise around the upper circle three times. Then move your hands, still in position one, to below your left rib and circle in the opposite direction three times around the upper circle.

For the lower belly: Begin just above your right hip bone, in line with the middle of your right thigh. Stroke up and across your belly button (right to left), down towards your left hip, cross back above the lower abdomen (left to right), then end above your right hip. Circle three times.

Knee to knee: Place your palms, one on top of the other, above your right knee. Make one big stroke up your right thigh all the way up to your lowest right rib, then go across to your left rib (right to left) and down the left side, pass your left hip and go down your left thigh to above your left knee. Repeat three times.

To end: Separating your hands again, put your right hand on your right thigh, palm down, and your left hand on your left thigh. Just rest your hands and softly inhale and exhale three times with your eyes closed.

FOOD IS POWERFUL SELF-CARE

'One cannot think well, love well, sleep well, if one
has not dined well.' *Virginia Woolf*

Feeding yourself well is a very simple way to show yourself some love and care
every day. If you do one single thing for yourself from this book, take some
time to cook a delicious meal that makes you feel good and nourishes your body.

Shopping, prepping and cooking make for the most powerful form of self-love
and self-care. Katia has included some of her favourite recipes in this book, and
we hope you'll love them too.

You may be thinking, avocado on toast is about the most I can do when I get
home from work. Or, who's got time to cook every day? But we promise you,
make time to learn one new, simple, nourishing recipe a week and in a couple of
months you'll have a roster of staple dishes that make you feel amazing.

Just compare the difference in how you feel the next time you make something
wholesome from scratch with fresh ingredients to when you buy something
on the run.

Eating well helps you stay mentally well. It is important to care about what you
put into your body, too, because it affects not only you but those around you.
Don't think about just filling your empty stomach by grabbing something easy –
think about nourishing and loving yourself through food that does you good.

FOOD PLANNING FOR BEGINNERS

We'd all love to be able to get in from work and just throw together an incredible feast from the fabulous ingredients that just happen to be in the fridge, but the reality is often a little different. Someone has to buy the food and fill the fridge. And packing it with lots of pre-prepared ingredients without any planning can lead to a lot of expensive waste.

A much more sensible approach is to plan your meals. Then you always know you'll have good food available and won't end up chucking so much away.

If, like Nadia, this kind of food planning isn't for you, instead make sure you have a selection of nourishing staples in your fridge or cupboards so you can always put together a little something without too much effort.

Katia is a great planner, and this is how she decides on what she's eating across a week:

1. Get out your diary and see what's coming up. Are you out in the evenings? Look at the time you have available to prep and cook this week. Who are you feeding? What time will you eat? Can you cook double for lunch or dinner the next day?

2. Once you know how many meals you need to make, write your shopping list for the week ahead. Ordering the ingredients online is super easy if you're really busy, but if you've got the time, or want to see and feel the food before you buy it, go to the farmers' market or your local greengrocer and butcher armed with your list.

3. When you've bought your food, think about whether you can prep any of it straight away so it's ready for a busier day. You could cook up some quinoa or chickpeas and put them in the fridge or freezer ready to put together with fresh ingredients for a speedy meal. Or chop some vegetables so they're ready to be dipped into your homemade hummus.

KATIA'S PANTRY FAVOURITES

People might think that because I run a health food café I advocate being restrictive about what you eat. But, honestly, my belief is that everything is fine in moderation, and you'll definitely find dairy, meat and gluten in my kitchen at home!

So, instead of restricting your diet, why not think about adding some new ingredients to your shopping basket? I believe the only true superfoods are the ones that make you feel great, and you should learn to pay attention to your body to find for yourself how it reacts to different foods.

To get you started, here are a few ingredients that I like to have in the pantry for quick and easy recipes that really work for me and for my family. I'm not suggesting you go out and buy all of these at once, but why not try a few?

Spirulina powder: Spirulina is high in protein and vitamins, and just a spoonful stirred into a smoothie gives you a really nutritious hit. When my kids aren't keen on eating their greens I can always get a smoothie down them. The powder lasts for ages in the cupboard, and a little goes a long way.

Bee pollen: Bee pollen is considered a nutritionally complete food. Yes, it's expensive, but you don't need much, just a sprinkle in smoothies, on granola or over fruit.

Cacao nibs: These crunchy pieces of raw cacao bean are quite bitter on their own, but mixed into granola or cookies they add a delicious chocolatey kick without the need to add sugar.

Coconut oil: Great for cooking, and you can even use it as a moisturizer or hair mask!

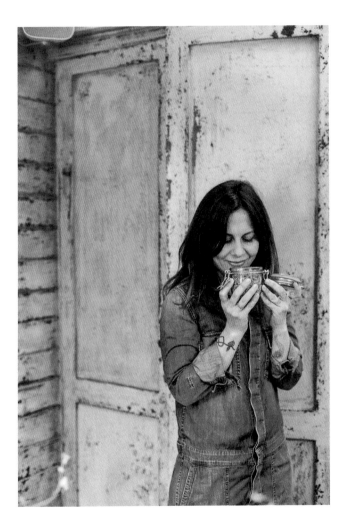

Quinoa: Most people are familiar with white quinoa, but I love to have a mix of red and black, too. It looks so pretty on the plate.

Chia seeds: Again, these are expensive, but they last a long time and you don't need to use much. They're full of protein and, because they swell in liquid, they add texture to puddings and smoothies.

Almond milk: I have cow's milk in my tea, but I also keep a few non-dairy milks to hand. Oat, almond and coconut milks are all delicious and because the boxed versions keep for ages, they're a great backup to have in the cupboard.

Frozen bananas: Rather than waste bananas that are going black, I like to peel and freeze them in ziplock bags. You can then chop them from frozen and add them to smoothies, or just whiz them up in the food processor to make a delicious, one-ingredient, banana ice cream.

Watercress: If I was going to urge you to add one thing to your diet from this whole list, it would be more leafy greens. Watercress happens to be my favourite, but try as many as possible.

Tahini: A staple ingredient for homemade hummus, and I also love to use it in dressings or drizzled over roasted vegetables.

Smoked paprika: This slightly spicy smoky powder will make any savoury recipe taste delicious – try it on hummus and cooked vegetables, and in salad dressings.

Almond butter: So versatile – try it in smoothies, salad dressings or on toasted sourdough, with a sliced banana, a sprinkling of cinnamon and a drizzle of honey.

Himalayan salt: This is the salt I use most often. It's more expensive than regular salt, but I love it because it's less processed and it is rich in minerals. Also, it's a really pretty pink colour!

EAT WHAT MAKES YOU FEEL GOOD

What's a self-care attitude to food? Eat what you want to eat. That doesn't mean eating everything indiscriminately, rather it's about eating the food your body needs at that moment. This is a good time to check into your wants and needs again, which we discussed in the introduction. Your body might want the whole packet of biscuits at once, but is that really what it needs?

Try to cultivate a calmness around what you feed yourself, and resist being too restrictive or giving yourself a hard time about what you're eating.

When we talk to most clients they often tell us, Oh, I need to give up sugar, or stop drinking coffee or eating chocolate or wheat. We really believe that a positive attitude to food doesn't mean restricting what you eat. Unless you have a medical condition, eating well doesn't have to mean gluten-free, sugar-free, dairy-free or 'clean eating'. We see a whole new wave of people who are obsessively healthy – we were once those people, too – but we've learned from experience that it's not so much about what you're eating as how you're eating it. Are you eating from a place of love and nourishment? Or out of punishment, or ideas of good and bad?

Being mindful of what you are eating and how it nourishes your body and your soul is a good start to practising self-care around food. Pay attention to how your body feels when you eat different foods – do you feel good afterwards? There may be a physical reaction from certain foods. Notice your energy levels; sugar and caffeine will give you a quick energy kick, but do you crash afterwards? When you eat something heavy, like a burger, do you feel tired afterwards? That's because your body needs the energy to digest, so it's making you slow down. Slowing down is fine if you have a quiet afternoon ahead, but not if you're going to be busy.

Your reactions to food are personal to you, and it's worth working them out. When you keep listening to your body, it will give you the signals you need.

EATING MINDFULLY

If you eat when you're upset or stressed or bored, you're not nourishing yourself – especially if you are eating to stuff down uncomfortable feelings like sadness or guilt. In this situation, not only are you probably not eating healthily, you're also unlikely to be chewing your food properly, so it will be hard to digest and you'll feel worse than ever.

Another kind of mindless eating is when you eat in front of the TV, or eat quickly while you are walking or driving.

If you want to learn to savour food and help your digestion do its job, ask yourself these questions:

* When and where do I eat mindlessly?

* When I do this, how am I feeling?

When you catch yourself eating this way, notice it, stop, and take a few deep breaths. Ask yourself:

* Do I need to keep eating this? Or have I had enough?

With your next bite, take time and effort to notice the flavours and textures of the food. Savour, enjoy and chew it, and let your body tell you when you are full.

When you make a habit of paying attention to mindless eating, you're already beginning to develop the habit of eating mindfully.

EATING FOR SELF-CARE

Although learning your own personal dietary needs is the most important thing, here are a few guidelines to help you make sure you are looking after your body and nourishing it properly.

* Cook and prepare as many different vegetables as you can get into every meal, especially for children. If your family like to eat meat, plan at least two vegetarian meals a week.

* Cook from scratch as often as you can manage. That way you know exactly what you're eating, with no hidden extras.

* Reduce your intake of processed or sugary food. That doesn't mean banning your children (or you) from crisps or sweets, but if you don't buy them, they're not in the cupboard for mindless snacking.

* Buy free-range and organic meat and dairy if you can. We like to get our fruit and vegetables from a local market or farmers' market where possible. It may cost a little bit more, but think of it as an investment in your health and a way of supporting the local community. If that's not an option for you, don't feel you've failed because you haven't lived up to some idealised version of yourself that's skipping round a farm carrying a wicker basket. Do what you can. It's about steps, not perfection.

* Know that sugar is sugar, whether it's in honey, maple syrup, rice syrup, malt or coconut sugar. We tend to cook with less-refined muscovado sugar, which contains a few extra nutrients, such as iron, potassium and magnesium, when compared to white sugar, but not enough to make it a health food!

* Make time to eat. So many of us catch ourselves just grabbing a sandwich on the run, or realise late in the day that we haven't eaten lunch. This is not self-care; this is living in fight and flight, so you're running on adrenaline and stressing out your digestive system.

MAKE MEALTIMES SACRED

Whether you're with people or on your own, make your mealtimes sacred. These rules may seem completely alien if you usually eat watching TV, reading or looking at a screen, but give it a try.

If you have a family and there's a rebellion brewing from your kids about you changing the way you eat, we suggest you try one meal a week, when you can all sit together and be your most relaxed – maybe Friday night dinner or Sunday lunch.

If you live on your own, try organising a regular dinner with your closest friends, the ones who are most like family, and maybe take it in turns to cook, so you are not always eating by yourself.

Remember, mealtimes should be fun, not just fuel.

* The table is a place to enjoy eating. This is the one time you can all be together, so treat it as the special time that it is. It is not the place to lecture a child (or an adult!) or raise a difficult subject for discussion.

* There should be no devices at the table – nor any books or newspapers either (though we make an exception at breakfast time).

* Eat home-cooked food when you can. This can be made by anyone in the family, of course, however young.

* Present the food nicely, whether you prefer it served in bowls in the middle of the table to share, or straight onto individual plates.

* Set the table nicely. It's a fun way to be creative.

* Talk about your day or week and get everyone else to do the same.

* Perhaps bring in a mealtime ritual: it could be saying thanks for the food, or raising glasses for a toast. Make it personal.

* Once a week, go round the table and give everyone a turn to say what they were grateful for that week.

* Make time for a relaxed meal, reminding children not to rush through their meal and to chew properly.

* Open your home to guests, maybe someone who doesn't have a family or doesn't live close to their family. It's always nice to feed people. Make their favourite dish, so they feel welcome.

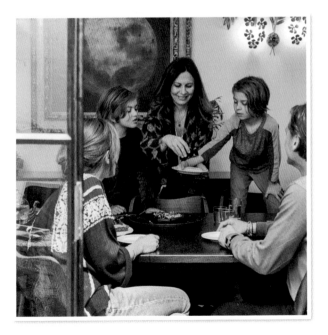

THE JOY OF EATING ALONE

If you're eating alone you might think it's not worth making an effort, but you can turn any meal into a moment of self-care that will help you appreciate the experience, and appreciate yourself. Treat yourself like your own guest!

* Put on some music and turn the preparation and cooking into something enjoyable and fun. Even if you're throwing together a salad, make a really satisfying dressing for it. If you're just having something on toast, add chopped herbs or a side salad. Imagine you were presenting this dish to someone you love – make it special.

* Put your food on a nice plate and arrange it beautifully. It doesn't need to be Instagram-worthy (not everything you eat needs to be photographed) but it does need to look enticing. When you start feeling proud of what you've made and the fact that you've made it just for you, it will encourage you to prepare food for yourself more often.

* We admit some of the meals we eat alone are wolfed down at the kitchen counter in a hurry – not good self-care! Make a point of eating at the table, and chew slowly to give your digestion maximum chance of getting every bit of goodness. It's not always easy to sit quietly to eat, we know, but if you can manage it regularly it can become a good habit. If you want to watch TV or a movie while you eat, go ahead and do it, but preferably not something stressful or violent.

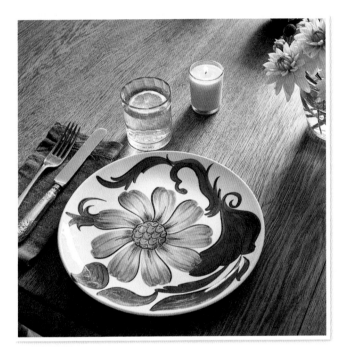

BEETROOT CHOCOLATE CAKE

*A deeply satisfying and moist chocolate cake with a touch
of earthiness from the iron-rich beetroot. This cake is so
well loved at the café that it's taken on a personality of
its own — we call it the Iron Maiden.*

Serves 8

200g butter

*200g dark chocolate
(70% cocoa), broken
into chunks*

*250g cooked vacuum-
packed beetroots
(the kind with
no vinegar)*

5 eggs

*250g coconut
sugar or light
muscovado sugar*

*1 tsp baking powder
(I use gluten-free
baking powder to
make this a
gluten-free cake)*

¼ tsp vanilla extract

240g ground almonds

pinch of salt

*dried rose petals, to
decorate (optional)*

Preheat the oven to 190°C/360°F/Gas mark 5 and line
a 20cm cake tin with baking parchment.

Melt the butter and chocolate in a glass bowl set
over a pan of gently simmering water, making sure the
bottom of the bowl doesn't touch the water. Once
melted, remove from the pan and leave to cool.

Blitz the beetroots to a purée in a food processor, then
add the eggs, sugar, baking powder and vanilla to the
bowl. Add the cooled chocolate and butter mixture
and pulse until mixed. Finally, add the ground almonds
and salt and pulse briefly to combine.

Pour this batter into the prepared cake tin and bake for
35–45 minutes. You'll know the cake is done because it
won't wobble when you take it out of the oven.

Don't worry if your cake has a crack on the top – it's
meant to look like that!

Sprinkle over the rose petals before serving, if you like.

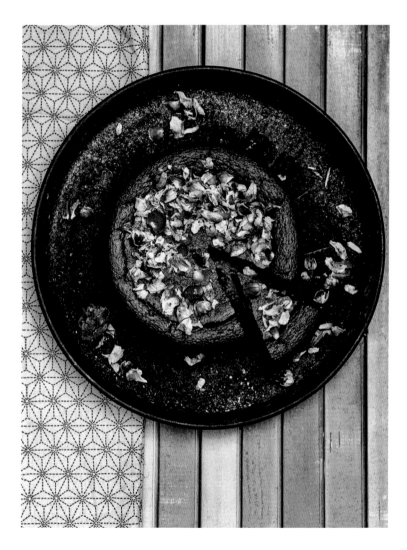

SALMON SKEWER WITH GREEK-STYLE RICE AND A YOGURT DRESSING

A super easy, quick lunch or supper to make when you've had a long day. Tell your fishmonger you're making skewers, because if the cubes are cut too small, they'll fall apart as they cook. If you're using salmon fillets from the supermarket, just slice the skin off with a sharp knife and cut them into cubes.

Makes 4 skewers

juice of 1 lemon

1 tbsp olive oil

2 garlic cloves, smashed and finely chopped

16 salmon cubes

1 courgette, sliced vertically, then into half moons

8 cherry tomatoes

½ onion, sliced vertically into three

salt and freshly ground black pepper

100g plain yogurt, to serve

First mix the lemon juice, olive oil and garlic together in a shallow bowl, then add the rest of the kebab ingredients and season with salt and pepper. Cover and leave to marinate in the fridge for 30 minutes.

While the fish marinates, put 4 skewers in water to soak and then get on with the rice. On a low heat, add the butter and olive oil to a pan and sauté the onion for 10–15 minutes until soft. Add the rice and let it sizzle for about 5 minutes so that each grain is coated in oil. Don't let the rice stick to the bottom of the pan.

Add the stock, cover the pan and bring to the boil. Once boiling, uncover the pan and turn down to a simmer. Cook for around 20 minutes (it will depend on your rice, so keep an eye on it), until the water has nearly all evaporated. Then turn off the heat, put the lid back on and let the rice sit and steam for 15 minutes.

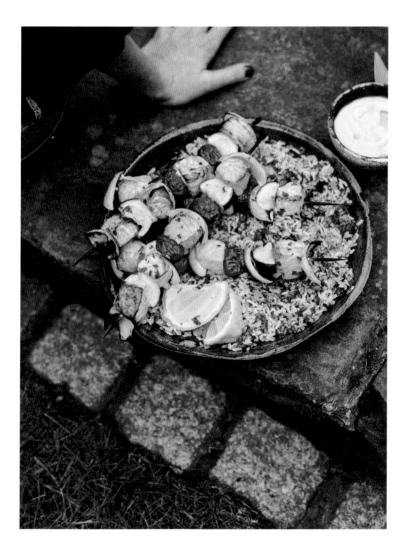

For the Greek rice
1 tbsp butter
1 tbsp olive oil
½ onion, finely chopped
200g rice (I use an easy cook brown rice)
500ml chicken or vegetable stock
small bunch of parsley, chopped
1 tbsp lemon juice

Heat the grill on high and line the grill tray with aluminium foil. Construct the skewers by threading the ingredients onto the soaked skewers, reserving the marinade to use later in the yogurt. I like to place 4 cubes of salmon, 4 pieces of courgette, 2 tomatoes and 3 slices of onion on each skewer.

Lay the skewers on the tray. The salmon will be mostly cooked from the marinade, so grilling them is just to finish them off and cook the vegetables, and perhaps get them a little charred. Put the skewers under the grill for 10 minutes, turning them twice or even three times to get them cooked evenly.

Heat up the leftover marinade until just boiling, then add it to the yogurt.

When the skewers are done, add the chopped parsley and lemon juice to the rice and stir it through. Plate up the rice, lay a skewer on top and let everyone help themselves to the yogurt sauce.

ROAST SWEET POTATO WEDGES
WITH POACHED EGGS

This is so pretty to look at, like golden sunshine on a plate. It's great for breakfast, lunch and dinner, as it's deeply satisfying and extremely simple to put together. It is perfect as it is but if you need a splash of green, try it with steamed spinach or Tenderstem broccoli on the side. If you're intimidated by poaching eggs, why not get a poaching pan? Or just fry them instead.

Serves 2

1 large sweet potato (500–600g), halved and cut into wedges

pinch of salt

salt and freshly ground black pepper

pinch of smoked paprika

olive oil, for drizzling

2 eggs

Preheat the oven to 190°C/360°F/Gas mark 5.

Put the sweet potato wedges on a baking tray and sprinkle over the salt, pepper, smoked paprika and olive oil. Massage all the ingredients into the sweet potato wedges until they are coated in the mixture, then roast in the oven for about 30 minutes, until soft and golden.

Ten minutes before the sweet potato is ready, get your eggs going. Boil the water in a poaching pan and grease the little egg holders with a little butter or olive oil. Crack the eggs into the pan and cook for about 3½ minutes, until the egg whites have become white and set but the yolk is still runny.

Arrange the sweet potato wedges in the middle of two plates, then slide your eggs on top. Drizzle with olive oil, scatter over a pinch of salt and dash of pepper and get stuck in!

Serves 4

bunch of watercress
(approx. 100g)

100g sunflower seeds

80g Parmesan cheese,
grated

½ bunch of basil
(approx. 10g)

3 tbsp chilli oil (if you
don't have chilli oil,
just add ¼ fresh red
chilli)

juice of 1½ lemons

¼ tsp salt

1 garlic clove, roughly
chopped

sprinkle of black
pepper

WATERCRESS PESTO

*I love this because it's super healthy and delicious. It's
not just for pasta; use it with courgetti or spiralised sweet
potato, or whack it on some toast or halves of roasted
butternut squash.*

Put the watercress in the blender first, as it makes
blending easier, then add the other ingredients. Whiz
until it's the right consistency for you – add a little
more oil if necessary; I like a little bit of texture and
crunch to my pesto. Use at once, or store in an airtight
jar in the fridge for up to 3 days.

Makes approx. 200ml

60ml water

60ml olive oil

thumb-sized piece of
root ginger, peeled
and roughly chopped

1 garlic clove, peeled
and roughly chopped

½ red chilli, deseeded
and roughly chopped

2 tbsp white miso

bunch of basil (approx.
25g)

1 tsp maple syrup

juice of 1 lime

WILD GREEN DRESSING

*We've tried this with other kinds of miso, but they can be
pretty salty, so at the café we stick to sweet white miso.
This dressing is great with salads, quinoa and all vegetables.*

Put everything into a blender and whiz until smooth.
Use at once, or store in an airtight jar in the fridge for
up to 4 days.

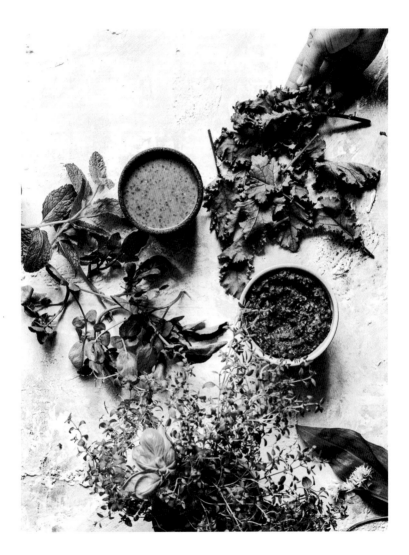

BUILDING YOUR RESOURCES

Think of your self-care like a savings account. When we are saving we try to put a small amount away every month for a rainy day or an emergency. In the same way, doing a little bit of self-care regularly will add up.

When you've got lots of time and energy it's a great opportunity to fill up your body bank account a bit more and increase the interest rate by doing good things for yourself. Putting good things in your self-care bank is how you build your resources, so that when life feels overwhelming – whether that's everyday things like city living, stress, tiredness or bigger situations when we are using every part of ourselves – you will always have some self-savings as a resource.

Think about what you did with the last spare 30 minutes you had. Did you spend it internet window shopping for things you don't need, or scrolling through Instagram? These sorts of activities won't give you many savings in the self-care bank.

If you're zoning out to back-to-back episodes of Real Housewives of Wherever, you're going into the self-care red zone, but if you're watching a show you absolutely love that makes you smile, laugh or cry … now you're getting closer.

It's even better to do something that makes you feel good in a deeper way. Look after yourself by connecting with people, or being creative or learning something new, or giving to someone in need. This is resourcing. This is filling yourself, your soul – and your self-care bank – from the inside out.

So how does self-care work in real life? Perhaps it's a Friday night, you're exhausted, you've had a long week at work and you're going to a party because it's your friend's birthday. You know it would mean a lot to them if you were there.

Maybe your usual habit is to start drinking straight after work, to give yourself the energy to get through the evening. Instead, see if you can organise your time beforehand, to give you a chance to take a nap for 20 minutes. Maybe you can go to the party later? If you can't take a nap, then perhaps have a nice long bath. If you can't do that, lie down for five minutes. What you need is a little rest, slotted between commitments, to refuel yourself.

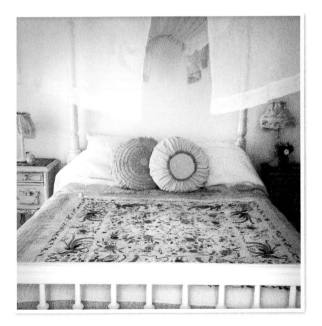

WHAT'S ON YOUR LIST OF RESOURCES?

To keep that self-care bank of resources in the black, think about what makes you feel good, what works for you, and make your own list of actions that leave you feeling relaxed, contented, rested or your best self. These are just some examples that work for us.

* Get to bed by 10.30pm (okay, 11pm!). Getting to bed early most nights and at around the same time will help you get your best sleep.

* Make some time each week to be sociable outside work with your easiest, most relaxed and positive friends, so you can totally be yourself.

* Move your body. Find a physical exercise you really, really enjoy so it doesn't feel as if you're having to work at it.

* A nap. If you can do this in the middle of the day, you're onto a winner. Put your phone on airplane mode, get out your softest blanket and curl up on the sofa for 20 minutes (or longer if you're lucky!).

* A long, luxurious bath with relaxing essential oils. Choose rose or frankincense oil for luxury, lavender for calming, bergamot or mandarin to uplift you.

* Live in the present. If your thoughts constantly drift off to what you've got to do tomorrow, next week or next month, you'll stress yourself out.

* Don't take things personally. If you do, you will exhaust yourself thinking, why did they say this? Or, how could they have done that? But know this: people do all kinds of things because of what is going on in their life. You may never find out their reasons, but they very likely have nothing to do with you.

* Do difficult things to make yourself proud. Everything is scary when you are doing it for the first time, whether it's having a kid, starting a business or just getting up in front of people to talk. If something challenges you, channel the title of the classic 80s self-help book, *Feel The Fear And Do It Anyway.* You'll feel amazing if you nail it, and if you don't, at least you bloody tried.

DIARISE YOUR SELF-CARE

Make self-care a priority by writing it, in pen, into your diary or planner. You don't have to start with one thing a day (though that'd be ideal), just choose three or four things that you can put into your week.

Instead of trying to eliminate things you don't want to do, add new, loving habits and let the good things grow. It could be as simple as getting an early night or as short as a five-minute meditation. Everyone's got five minutes, and it's a great place to start.

The more you do of the stuff that feels good, the more you'll feel good, and the more you're going to want to do the good stuff. It's a virtuous circle.

SELF-CARE IN UNDER FIVE MINUTES

If you're lucky enough to have longer than five minutes, of course you can do all of these exercises for longer. Set an alarm for the time you have available and really let yourself get into it, even if you feel a bit silly at first.

* Shake it up. Standing up, bend your knees a little and start doing a light bounce, keeping both feet on the ground. Stretch your arms up over your head, shake out your wrists, still lightly bouncing through your knees. Shake out your right wrist, then your whole right arm. Shake out your left wrist, then your whole left arm. Shake your right ankle, then your whole right leg, your left ankle, then your whole left leg, then begin to shake out your whole body.

* Dance to one of your favourite songs. Just close your eyes and get moving, and hope no one is watching! Even if they are, who cares?

* Try this calming breath. Breathe in for four counts, then out for four. Breathe in for four and increase the exhalation to six, then breathe in for four and increase your exhalation to eight counts.

* Just sit. Relax back in a chair so your body is really resting, and close your eyes. Pay attention to the parts of your body that are tense. See if you can breathe into them to relax them.

* Try dry skin brushing; it is super energising and great for the lymphatic system, which boosts your immunity. Do this before your shower in the morning. You do need a special skin brush, but they sell them in most chemists. Brush your body in circular motions, then sweep brush strokes towards the heart. If you don't have a brush, you can make claws with your hands and use your fingertips instead. Apply firm pressure up your legs, arms and body, always going towards the heart.

* Read a few pages of an inspirational book. Keep a pile of books next to your bed, on a table by your favourite chair, or even on your desk, so you can pick one up when you need a bit of inspiration and just read a few paragraphs or pages. They should be books that make you feel joyful, nothing to do with duties, work or being a parent.

* Get outside in nature, even if it's just a patch of grass between buildings. Look up at the sky. Take a few deep breaths.

* Try a five-minute simple meditation. Sit quietly and pay attention to your breath. Notice when your mind wanders and just come back to your breath. See how calm and centred you feel afterwards – this could be the start of a beautiful meditation habit.

* Rest in the dark. Set your alarm for however much time you need, lie down on your bed, close the curtains and put on a sleep mask to block out all light. Then just rest.

* Take a fast shower. Sprinkle a few drops of your favourite essential oil onto the floor of the shower, so as the warm water hits it, the scent surrounds you. Peppermint is a good uplifting and mind-clearing oil.

HOW TO MAKE A GOOD HABIT

We all want to develop good habits, the ones that will serve us and care for us effortlessly. You probably don't have to force yourself to brush your teeth every morning – it's just a habit you do without thinking. The more good habits we can do automatically, the better we feel. In the Kundalini yoga tradition, it's believed you can heal your habits by doing something daily. They believe that:

In 40 days, you can break a negative habit.

In 90 days, you can establish a new habit.

In 120 days, you will ingrain that new habit.

In 1000 days, you will master the new habit.

Here's how to use that process. First, choose what your new habit or self-care practice will be. Will it be a little bit of yoga every day, or meditation, or turning off your phone earlier in the evening?

Whatever you decide, make a calendar on a piece of squared paper – give yourself 40 days, or 90 or even 120 – with a little square for each day.

When you have completed your habit each day, mark a square with a tick. See how you feel after 40 days. Make a note, keep going, and see if you notice a difference after 90 days, and so on.

Soon enough your good things will grow and you'll notice the difference between what feels good and what doesn't.

You don't have to struggle for change. Once you start paying attention, you'll find change can happen naturally.

Nadia: 'For years I tried to give up my (very) part-time social smoking. It was my last vice, just the odd cigarette with a friend or at a party. Before a party, I'd tell myself, "I won't smoke. How can I smoke? I'm a yoga teacher, for God's sake. Yoga teachers don't smoke!" I knew I didn't actually enjoy the taste or the smell or the regret afterwards, but I'd always have one because it felt fun and cool and naughty.

'So I stopped "trying" not to smoke. Instead, I started to pay attention to how a cigarette tasted, how my body felt afterwards, how my skin looked the next day.

'With that new perspective, the next time I had a cigarette, I saw myself from the outside. I thought about what it was doing to my insides. And both images were gross. I realised I just could not smoke one more cigarette. Now it's been three years, and I haven't even wanted to smoke. I was ready.'

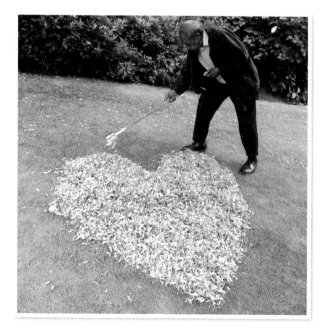

HOW TO GROW
MORE LOVE
IN YOUR LIFE

* Check in with yourself. Notice how you feel. Do this every day, a few times a day if you can.

* Ask yourself, what does love feel like to you? Not just romantic love, but love for others, the planet, yourself.

* When do you feel you are not aligned with the feeling of love?

* Ask yourself, what would loving and caring for myself feel like right now in this moment?

* What could you do, right now, to feel more love in your life?

* Do something loving for yourself today.

hope

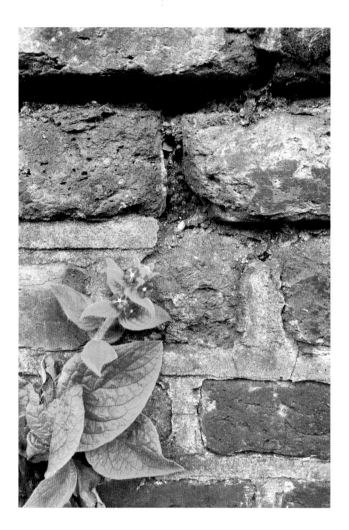

> "I learned that when life pulls you under, you can kick back
> against the bottom, break the surface and breathe again.'
> *Sheryl Sandberg*

It's easy to be hopeful and happy when everything's going well in your life, but no amount of positive thinking, or even self-care, can save you from times when things just feel a bit crap.

When you're faced with these moments, big or small, remind yourself that struggling doesn't mean you've failed, it just means you're human.

The truth is, the perfect life doesn't exist for anyone – not even that person you follow on Instagram who seems to have it all together. Your life doesn't need to be perfect to be a life you can love. Once you know that, you can stop waiting for things to reach some unlikely ideal and get on with enjoying the life you have right now.

We hope these chapters will help you find your potential, to grow and change and become more you. Isn't that worth being hopeful about?

COMPARISON

'Comparison is the thief of joy.' *Theodore Roosevelt*

Comparing yourself to others is a normal, human impulse. When you're feeling good about yourself it can even inspire you to make positive changes in your own life. But generally it's healthier to stick to your own path and not look around too much. Comparison becomes magnified by a million on social media, and too much of it can eat away at your own sense of self-worth. Good things can come from social media, of course – it's a way to stay connected to people and ideas, and it can inform and inspire you – but it needs careful handling.

Maybe you've got a habit of getting online first thing in the morning, before you've even got out of bed? Or maybe you're sitting online for hours on a Sunday night, looking at other people's lives, checking out their weekends. What is she doing? Where is he? Why wasn't I invited?

Try to remember that what you're looking at online is other people's edited highlights. You're comparing their carefully curated photographs and words with your complicated, beautiful, scrambled human mess of reality. We all know this but we can't help ourselves scrolling through other people's feeds, judging them and deciding that they have more than us; that their lives are perfect.

After a session on Instagram or Facebook, think about how you feel. Inspired? Grateful? Happy with your own life? Or, more likely, not. Try to be aware of how time spent online affects your emotions. Some therapists even refer to too much time online as a form of self-harm.

WHAT'S THE STORY?

You never know what somebody else's story is. People can have so much going on on the outside and yet be miserable on the inside. Even people who seem to have everything – career success, a huge house, a loving family, all the possessions they desire – can feel like they're missing something. Everyone is searching for meaning or purpose in their lives in some way, even if it doesn't seem like it to those around them.

On social media, looking at someone's exterior image, you've got no idea what they're dealing with. You're comparing their outsides to your insides. You don't know if their kid had a tantrum after the adorable picture was taken, or if the yogi makes that impossible position look so effortless because she's a professional dancer who started training at the age of three.

You don't know the sheer organisation or the number of photographs it took to get that perfectly casual walking-down-the-street picture, or how much of the real moment they may have missed by styling it so carefully.

But we all still look at that picture, and judge ourselves to be lacking: not talented enough, not pretty enough, not rich enough, not popular enough, not happy enough. It doesn't help that we're often looking at social media in a quiet moment, maybe while travelling or sat at home. When our own lives are busy and full, we don't have time to go down the online rabbit hole.

Comparison happens in real life, too. You've just screamed at your kids trying to get them out of the door in the morning, then you arrive at school to see The Perfect Mum laughing with her children, and you hate and judge yourself and think you are a terrible mother. Or your best friend tells you her amazing news, she's pregnant – again! – and you feel devastated because you're not even in a relationship.

At least when you see someone face to face you get the experience of the person and potentially the opportunity to find the real story. On social media, you can't get to the other side of the picture – it's available 24/7 and often you don't even know the people you are looking at.

> Nadia: 'Once a friend commented on an Instagram picture of me dressed up in a great outfit at a friend's party. Because she was feeling a bit vulnerable, she assumed I was having an incredible time and my entire life was amazing. Meanwhile, the truth is, I didn't have a great night and was home in bed by 10.30pm!'

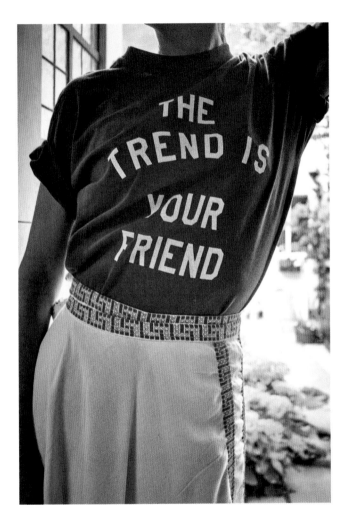

SELF-CARE FOR SOCIAL MEDIA

* Choose carefully who you follow. Don't look at posts or people that you know trigger your insecurities. Can you cut your follows down to close friends and inspiring people?

* Don't look at social media first thing, and not after 8pm. Evenings are a vulnerable time when your emotions can become magnified. Give yourself a break.

* If you're in a low place, limit social media. Like drinking, it's not wise to do it when you're sad.

* Be mindful how you feel about people before you look them up. Don't look at any exes where the relationship isn't mended, or anyone you've fallen out with, or a friend who's not being a good friend to you right now. The story you're telling yourself – she's got perfect children, he's got a beautiful new girlfriend who's younger than me – is not about them, it's your creation, about what that person represents to you.

* Be responsible with your own posts. Do them to inspire and interest people, not to impress anyone or to prove yourself, or to make a point.

* Take conscious phone breaks.

* Switch off notifications, so that you engage with social media on your own terms, instead of being bombarded by it.

* No phones when you're eating. But you knew that, right?

* Followers are not friends. Don't confuse the two.

Katia: *'Since I got my dog, Batman, I go for a walk every day for an hour, purposefully leaving my phone at home. It's so I can enjoy being in the moment, and not document the moment instead. It allows me to check in with how I'm feeling and it can be a moment to be creative. If I'm stressed or angry, that time alone gives me space to respond, rather than react, to calm down before I have to deal with people.'*

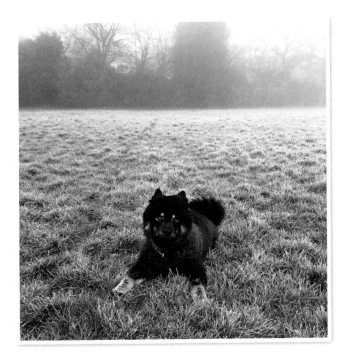

INFUSED WATER

Here are some ideas for a few of my favourite infused waters. They are so simple to make. It's best to infuse your water for about 30 minutes before you drink it. Once it's made, keep it in the fridge and try to use it up within 12 hours.

Fill a jug with filtered water and add one of the following:

Sliced lemon + sliced lime + mint leaves = vitamin boost

Strips of cucumber + mint leaves + sliced watermelon = refresh

Sliced orange + sliced grapefruit + rosemary sprigs + cinnamon sticks = warming

Sliced strawberries + mint leaves + rose water = mood boost

Sliced pineapple + lime + mint = digestion

Lemon + ginger = cleanse

CRYSTAL WATER

The crystal waters at the Nectar Café were designed for us by Michael Isted from The Herball. The idea behind them is, the water is charged by the crystals, taking on the vibrations and properties of the healing crystals. You can do this at home using the crystal that resonates most with you.

Obviously you are only going to be attracted to this if you believe in the power of crystals, but I urge you to try it even if you don't. Next time people are over for dinner and you have a water jug on the table, add a few crystals – it will look beautiful.

Here are some crystals you can use, and their healing properties:

Citrine – manifesting abundance (add a drop of orange blossom water)

Amethyst – promotes peacefulness and happiness (add a drop of lavender water)

Rose quartz – unconditional love (add a drop of rose water)

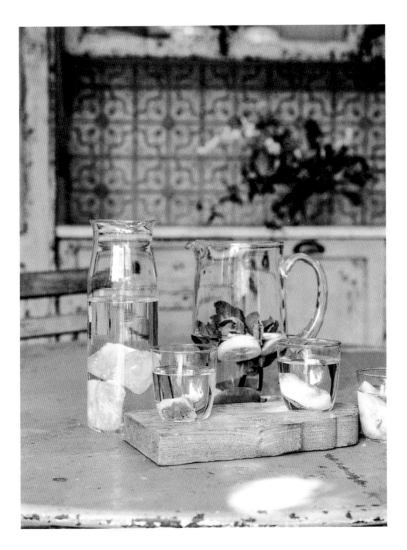

GRATITUDE: THE ANTIDOTE
TO COMPARISON

As a human being, you can choose to focus on what you have and not on what you don't have. Gratitude, the experience of counting your blessings and saying thank you for what you have, makes you learn to be happy with exactly what you've got.

Practising gratitude by consciously thinking of things you are grateful for, or writing them down, has a measurable and lasting effect on your brain. Studies suggest that actively practising gratitude can help you sleep better and leave you feeling less stressed, and that the effects can be long lasting.

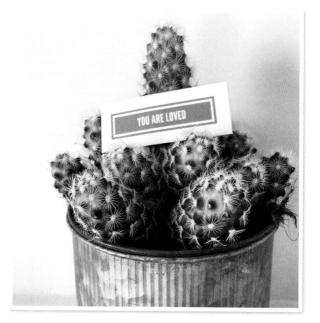

HOW TO CULTIVATE GRATITUDE
IN YOUR LIFE

* The simplest way is to think of three things you're grateful for while you're in bed, in those moments as you are waking up, or as you are falling asleep. Do this at night time and it can help you get to sleep. Do it in the morning and it will set up your day on a positive note.

* Write three things you're grateful for in a journal every day. Yes, it sounds kind of corny, we know, and of course you can just do it in your head like we suggested above, but we've found the great thing about writing it down is that these moments of gratitude are there for you to read all over again when things are feeling difficult.

* Write a letter of thanks to someone. Now that everything is digital, a real handwritten card or letter sent through the post is extra special.

* Say thank you to someone and really mean it. When people take the time to tell us they love the food at the Nectar Café, it makes us all feel amazing.

* Give good feedback. This is great to do on social media and can combat those feelings of comparison.

* Sit and talk at the dinner table with friends or family about the good things that have happened that day or week. Make every night – or maybe just every Sunday lunch – a little Thanksgiving meal.

* Make a note of things you're grateful for and collect them all together. Write the notes on colourful bits of paper and put them in a glass jar where you can see them. If you have kids, this exercise can help them to recognise good and bad feelings as well as what they're grateful for. You can do the opposite, too: some people like to write down anything that was bad in the day and then, before bed, they throw it in the bin or a fire to clear their heads.

SOLVING THE MONEY PUZZLE

Practising self-care around money can be difficult for a lot of people. It can be hard not to be consumed with worry or to find ourselves struggling with managing our finances or our debts.

Self-care means finding a healthy balance where you pay attention to money and respect it, but you don't let it define you. Of course, that's assuming you have enough money to cover your basic needs (and if you do, you're doing better than a lot of people in the world).

There are two basic types of money struggle. There's the person who is super frugal and doesn't like to spend at all; this person needs to learn to trust a little more that they will be okay if they loosen the reins of their spending. It helps to think of money as a form of energy that flows between people, not something always to hold on to. The good quality of frugal people is that they are aware of their financial situation and they know how to budget, which is a great start.

The other kind of person is someone who spends and spends without any concept of where the money is going. This person needs to give their money more respect – to think about spending with care and attention instead of splurging mindlessly. If this is you, try to write down everything you buy for a few weeks, or even a month, then look back over your purchases and think about why you bought them. Remember, you can't buy yourself peace or happiness.

When it comes to money and self-care, try to cultivate a good balance.

* Look at all you have and tell yourself, I am grateful for all I have. Gratitude and money should go hand in hand.

* Almost everyone can give a little to charity; in many religious traditions you give ten per cent of your income to good causes. Find a charity to support that moves you, and give what you can. If you can't give money, can you volunteer your time?

* Practising self-care around money means having clear and stated boundaries. Put in place what's going to happen before you lend someone money or share bills or expenses. And if you lend someone money, be prepared that you may not get it back!

* Be generous. It's always a wonderful trait, whether it's buying someone dinner or a gift. Generosity doesn't have to be big or expensive, just the gesture is always appreciated.

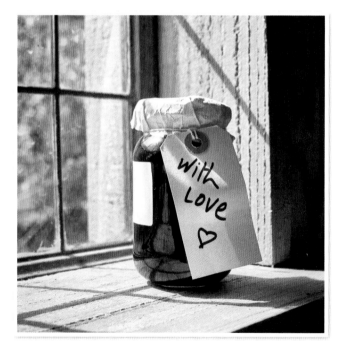

CONFIDENCE

*'I figure, if a girl wants to be a legend, she should go
ahead and be one.' Calamity Jane*

What was the last thing you said to yourself about yourself? 'I can't eat that because I'm too fat?' 'I can't do that because I've never done it before?' 'I can't say that because they'll think I'm stupid?' We are way more careful with what we say to other people than how we talk to ourselves. To ourselves, we can be so damn mean.

If you could only see yourself the way your best friend sees you, you would appreciate how beautiful, clever, funny and interesting you are.

It might feel like everyone else is more confident than you, but we can assure you, they're not! Believe us when we say there are beautiful, talented people who are universally admired and considered to be confident who present a very different front to the world to the nervousness they are feeling inside.

GROWING YOUR CONFIDENCE

Some people are fortunate to have confidence installed in their default settings by parents or loved ones. It is the ultimate gift. But if you weren't given it, you can find a way to it as an adult. You have to figure it out for yourself. We hope these tips will help.

* Do something that scares you. It could be making a speech, talking to a stranger at a party or trying a new hobby. The more you practise the things that feel scary, the less intimidating they become and the more confidence you will have for new challenges.

* Be you. Real confidence isn't just being the best at what you can do in your life, but being true to yourself. When you meet someone who is okay with being vulnerable and honest and open, you feel it instantly. That is so much more interesting than someone who puts on a mask. You can be successful at what you're doing professionally but if you're not being your true self, it won't feel right inside.

* Take care of yourself. Yes, we are going on about this, but the more care you take of yourself, the better you'll feel about yourself, and the more good you'll want to do in the world.

* If you are feeling stuck, ask a very wise friend for help, or possibly a life coach. Sometimes you need someone on the outside to spur you on and encourage you.

* When the scary thoughts creep in, telling you that you can't or shouldn't do something, notice this is happening. This is the first step to realising they're just thoughts! Then you will realise that you can change them.

IF YOU DON'T LIKE YOUR INNER VOICE, GET A NEW ONE

Pay attention to what you say to yourself about yourself. It's easy to get into the habit of self-criticism. It often goes something like this: I am not worthy, I am not enough, I am going to be laughed at or despised or looked down on or found out.

This isn't the real voice inside you. That voice is kind and loving, and if you can pay attention, you will find it. Self-criticism is simply an old thought pattern that's the opposite of self-care.

Every time you say something bad about yourself, something you wouldn't say to a friend, write it down. This will make you pay attention to how often you do it, so you can start to cut down this habit.

Oh, and it doesn't matter if you're being self-deprecating and trying to make people laugh. Even if you think you're being funny while you're putting yourself down, you're still eroding your confidence. You will start to believe what you say about yourself and in turn that creates your reality. Would you make someone else the butt of a joke by pointing out their flaws? If you wouldn't do that to someone else, don't do it to yourself.

Once you've written down your self-critical thought or what you said, think, what could you say about yourself differently? What can you say that's good instead?

Don't worry, this isn't bragging. Telling yourself good things about yourself is not the same as crowing to others about how fabulous you are. Those people who crave recognition from the outside are often the least confident on the inside.

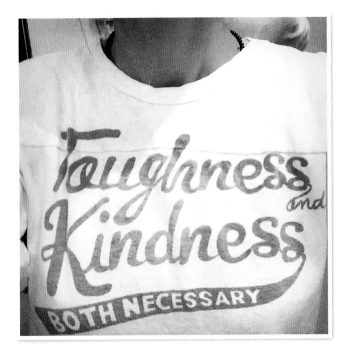

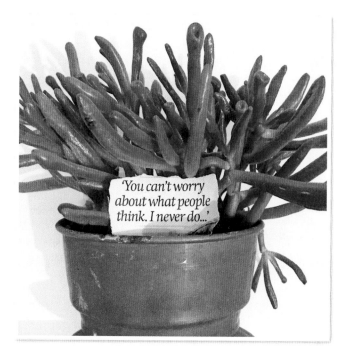

THE POWER OF POSITIVE QUOTES

Affirmations were big in the 80s. You were supposed to stick a note saying, for example, 'I love myself', on your mirror and, despite it being a bit cringey if anyone else saw it, it would change how you felt.

Affirmations have moved on since then, though. The change is subtle: the affirmation that works is the one you can believe. So, 'I love myself' won't work for everyone, but 'I am learning to love myself' may. If you want to try using affirmations, find one you can really believe in and repeat it to yourself every day, or write it down somewhere you will see it regularly.

An alternative to affirmations is reading and repeating quotes from great thinkers. These can be truly inspirational and can really change the way you think and feel. You might find some of these quotes super cheesy, and that's okay. Just keep looking until you find one that resonates with you.

When you find a quote that means something to you, write it on a post-it and stick it on your mirror, your keyboard or at your desk, even on your screen saver. Share them, too; when our poet friend Vinny visits, he leaves short poems and positive sayings in the most random places, such as under a pillow or in the bathroom cabinet, so his friends will find them long after he's left.

> Nadia: 'I tried a trick from Sophia Amoruso, author of #Girlboss: to change my password to an affirmation. I chose: IloveNadia. And every time I put my password in, it made me smile. Until my computer broke and I had to give the Mac guy my password! Mortifying.'

HOW TO ENVISION YOUR LIFE
WITH MOOD BOARDS

If you want a particular change to happen in your life, you need to direct it. You wouldn't just get in a car and drive without having any idea where you are going. Think of this mood board technique as your sat nav; it concentrates your intentions to help you head in the right direction. Mood boards or mood books can sound complicated and time consuming but, we warn you, once you start, they're addictive – you won't want to stop.

You can create a mood board, or a mood book, for your life in general, or for one specific part of it, such as your home, work or relationship, your future hopes, dreams and wishes, or what you'd like for your children.

Katia did a board for the launch of her café and she uses them regularly for dinner plans and kids' party themes. Nadia got heavily into Pinterest when she was doing up her house, staying up until 2am to pin inspiration onto her mood boards to help her create her dream home.

The lo-fi way

Cut out photos, words, quotes, sketches from magazines, whatever feels right to build the life vibe you'd like. Think about goals and meanings. Arrange your images and words on a board or in a scrapbook. You might want to put these images on a wall that people don't see when they come into the house, if you don't want to share it, or paste it to the inside of a cupboard door. The more private it is, the more you can go for it.

The online way

As you likely know, you can create folders for all the different areas of your life in Pinterest, and you can even print them if that helps. You'll find so many people to follow, with loads of creative ideas to inspire you. It's super fun and a brilliant way to create moods for any area of your life.

FOMO

(AND ITS OPPOSITE, JOMO)

'Enjoy life as it is and loving yourself as you are.' Kate Crow

Are your thoughts ever like this? 'Everyone else is there and I'm not.' 'Everyone is having fun, and I'm not.' 'I'm missing out.' 'I'm the only one who's alone and lonely.'

No matter who you are, there will always be someone who's having bigger, better, further flung, sexier, more exotic, more expensive, better-looking, more famous-friend-filled fun than you. Although it stings, FOMO (Fear Of Missing Out) may be giving you a message that you need to change something in your own life. What are all those other people doing that you're craving? Do you need to force yourself to say yes more often – maybe to go on a date, to get yourself to yoga class, to do the things you long to do?

The ultimate self-care is to do exactly what you feel like at that moment. If staying home is what you need, that's fine. But don't stay in looking at social media, wondering about what everyone else is doing. That will just deplete you.

You could also embrace JOMO. The Joy Of Missing Out is feeling the true delight of being on your own, of being able to watch the movie you want to, to take a bath and do exactly as you like.

Pay attention to yourself and know what your capacity for socialising is, in the moment. If you have plenty of energy and you feel good, get yourself out there and make the most of it. There will be times when you don't have much energy, or maybe the other parts of your life are full and you need some downtime. That's when you can really embrace JOMO.

HOW TO SOCIALISE HAPPILY

(especially if you're not feeling super social)

One way to make sure you have a good time when you go out is to work out exactly what a good time is for you.

* Think about the social events you've enjoyed most: how many people were there? Do you prefer one-on-one dinners or groups of 20? Pay attention to how things feel to you. Once you know the kind of scale you like, you can organise your social life to fit. It's good to be clear if you don't enjoy big dinner parties, otherwise you can end up being hard on yourself when you go and don't have fun.

* Do you hate big parties with loads of people you don't know? It doesn't mean you can't like them. You might find you prefer to go with someone you really like and engage in the experience with them. Or if the music is good, maybe you can lose yourself on the dance floor?

* If you haven't done the activity before – say a daytime rave, a bowling evening, karaoke – remember sometimes it's good to say yes to invitations. You might just have a brilliant time. Don't say no because you're scared.

* Don't get in the habit of always staying in. There's a difference between taking some time out for yourself (good) and retreating from the world (not so good). Sometimes you have to make yourself do things, otherwise people can stop inviting you – and you might regret that.

* If socialising takes a lot out of you, make sure you've got time to recover afterwards.

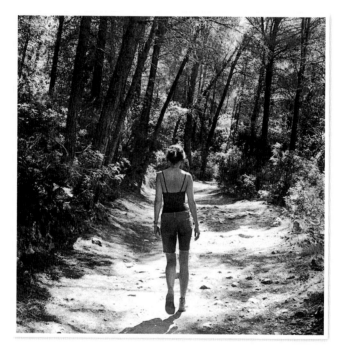

HOW TO BE ON YOUR OWN

(especially when you don't want to be)

Time by yourself resources you. Learn to enjoy your own company and let go of ideas of being embarrassed or ashamed about being on your own. Even if you're an extrovert and always need to be around people, it's important to know how to be by yourself.

Maybe you don't like solitude because your thoughts become loud and it feels as if there's too much going on in your head. Take a leap and stay with the discomfort. You will eventually become more familiar with it and it won't seem so weird.

If you practise being on your own, you will learn to be okay on your own, and this will be a source of strength for the rest of your life. You can't rely on someone else always being there to make you feel good, whether that's a partner of 25 years or your kids.

* If you find you have a night coming up with nothing planned, try not to fill the space. Book the time out for you, alone.

* Plan a delicious meal. Make it something you wouldn't usually cook just for you.

* Do the things you prefer not to do in front of someone else. Maybe this is a good time to create your mood board. Read a book or magazine you've been looking forward to. Try not to waste the evening zoning out to trashy TV.

* Don't do the housework/washing/ironing/accounts. Make the effort not to answer emails or do admin. Time out from socialising doesn't have to be filled with activity to be worthwhile.

QUINOA AND WILD RICE SALAD

Dried barberries might be tricky to find, unless you have a Middle Eastern shop near you, but it's worth trying to get them online, as they add a unique and deliciously tart hit to this salad. If you can't get hold of any, you can replace them with dried cranberries.

Serves 4

100g wild rice

100g quinoa (I like to use a mix of red, white and black)

1 corn on the cob

3 tbsp olive oil

1 spring onion, finely chopped

1 garlic clove, crushed

100g Tenderstem broccoli, chopped into bite-sized pieces

3 tbsp dried barberries or dried cranberries

juice and zest of 1 lemon

salt and freshly ground black pepper

1 red chilli, deseeded and finely chopped

30g toasted pumpkin seeds

Add the rice and quinoa to a saucepan and cover with about 5cm of water. Bring to the boil then turn the heat to the lowest setting and let simmer for 20 minutes, or until the water is nearly evaporated. Once the water is almost gone, try the rice – if it's undercooked, add a little more water, but if it's al dente, just turn off the heat and cover with a lid.

While the quinoa and rice sits, heat a frying pan until extremely hot. Char the corn in the dry pan, rotating it so that it's blackened in spots all over. Allow to cool.

Add 1 tablespoon of the olive oil to a pan and sauté the spring onion and garlic on a low heat for a couple of minutes, then add the broccoli for a few minutes. You want it to still have a crunch and be green, so don't overcook it.

Once the corn is cool enough to handle, take a sharp knife and slice the kernels off the cob.

In a large bowl, mix everything together with the barberries, lemon juice and zest, and the rest of the olive oil. Sprinkle over the chopped chilli and the pumpkin seeds, then season with salt and pepper.

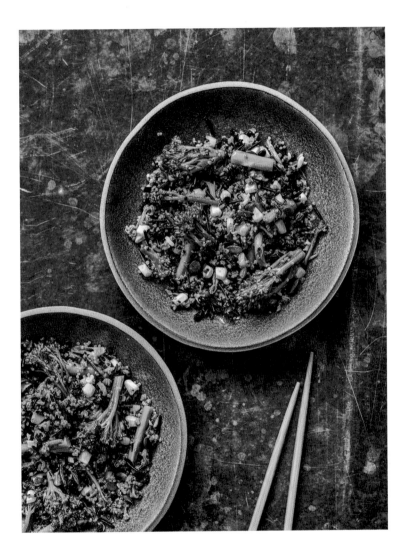

VEGETABLE KORMA

*thumb-sized piece of
root ginger (approx.
50g), peeled and
roughly chopped*

*3 garlic cloves, roughly
chopped*

*1 red chilli, deseeded
and roughly chopped*

1 tbsp coconut oil

1 onion, finely chopped

2 tsp ground cumin

1 tsp ground turmeric

½ tsp ground coriander

½ tsp ground cinnamon

*2 x 400g tins of
coconut milk*

1 vegetable stock cube

½ tsp salt

1 tbsp flour

*1 small butternut
squash (approx.
650g), peeled and
roughly chopped*

*1 cauliflower (approx.
350g), broken
into florets*

*100g mangetout or
sugar snap peas*

*1 big handful of
cavolo nero or
kale, chopped*

juice of 1 lime

*Don't be put off by the long list of ingredients, this is a
really easy curry to make. It lasts for three days in the
fridge and it freezes really well, too. A traditional korma
uses cream, but I've replaced it here with coconut milk.*

Whiz the ginger, garlic and chilli in a food processor
until finely chopped. Set aside.

Heat the coconut oil in a medium saucepan on a low
heat. Add the chopped onion and sauté until soft,
making sure it doesn't brown. Then add the ginger and
chilli mix and sauté for a minute, while stirring.

Now add your spices and stir for a minute to combine,
then pour in the coconut milk, stock cube and salt and
give it all a good stir to combine. Bring it to a simmer.
Meanwhile, combine the flour with 3 tablespoons of
water to make a thick paste, then add to the simmering
coconut milk.

Add the butternut squash, cook for 10 minutes, then
add the cauliflower and simmer for a further 10–15
minutes. Once you can pierce the vegetables with a
knife, throw in the mangetout and cavolo nero or kale
and cook for just 1 minute so they stay a vibrant green.

Take off the heat and squeeze in the lime juice.

Serve with boiled or steamed brown rice and sprinkle
with coconut flakes and toasted cashews.

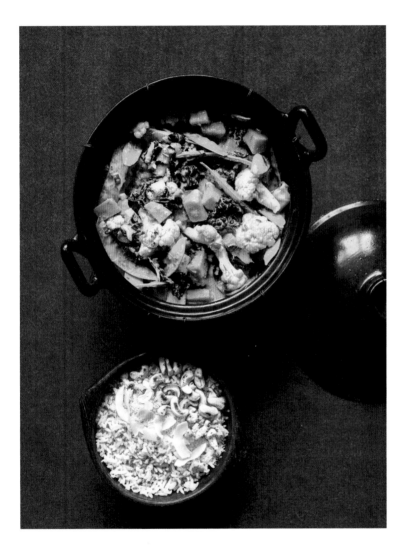

GOLDEN TURMERIC LATTE

At the Nectar Café, we're proud to make our latte mix using fresh root instead of powdered turmeric. Fresh mix gives a great anti-inflammatory boost, and the ingredients are also supposed to improve brain function and aid digestion. Pepper enables the absorption of the curcumin in the turmeric. Long pepper is worth seeking out, but you could use black pepper if you can't find it. The recipe makes 150ml of mix, which you can either use for making up lattes (2 tablespoons at a time), or take daily as a 15ml shot.

75ml ginger juice (from 150–200g ginger root, depending on your juicer)

75ml turmeric juice (from approx 130g turmeric root)

¼ tsp ground long pepper

Mix the ginger and turmeric juice with the long pepper powder. Transfer to a bottle and store in the fridge for up to 4 days.

To make 1 latte

200ml milk (I use oat milk)

2 tbsp golden latte mix

1 tsp maple syrup (optional)

sprinkle of ground cinnamon (optional)

Warm the milk in a pan, pour in the golden latte mix and stir to combine. You can use some maple syrup if you like a sweeter flavour, and serve the drink topped with a dusting of cinnamon.

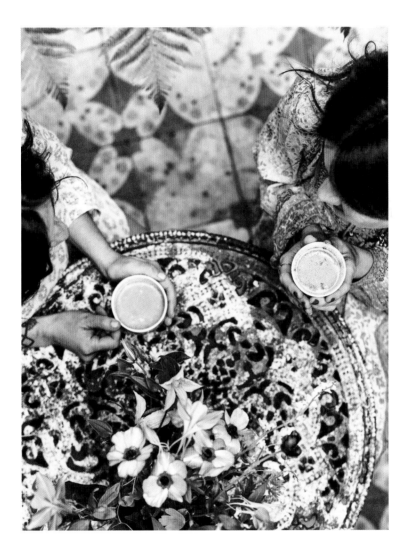

WHEN LIFE ISN'T PERFECT

'Everything can be taken from a man but one thing: the last of the human freedoms – to choose one's attitude in any given set of circumstances.' *Viktor Frankl*

So you don't have the relationship you wanted or expected. Or the child or children. Or the job. Or the castle with a moat on top of a hill. Life isn't perfect. It may not even come close.

So what happens next? Are you going to spend your life waiting for something to happen for you to be happy – maybe a lottery win, or to be rescued by a romance? What if those things never happen for you? When are you going to let yourself be happy?

Regardless of your situation, your life is precious and it has purpose right now, as it is. You deserve to wake up every day with a sense of joyfulness. The good news is, no matter where you start from you can get to a place of being comfortable with who you are. Find the things that fill you up and do the things that give you joy: seeing your friends, going to work, anything that makes you feel good.

When you make this decision, to be happy now and act on it, you will think less about the things you don't have.

COMPROMISE IS NOT A BAD WORD

There are times in your life when you have to be flexible and compromise. And that isn't always a bad thing. If you have been on your own with only yourself to answer to and suddenly you are in your dream relationship, there may be things your new beau may want to do (or not) and you will find you have to compromise a bit.

No one is perfect, not everyone is exactly like you (thank God) and life doesn't happen exactly as you would like it to. So being flexible is a quality we all need to learn for any relationship to work – whether that's a romantic one or one with a friend or colleague.

You also have to compromise because no one person can do everything they want to do. Different needs will take priority at various times in your life: children, illness, work, where you live, your relationship. It all needs to be juggled and balanced, so it cannot be perfect, but if you can embrace it you'll find the perfection in that imperfection.

> Katia: 'I've been offered investment to build my business, the Nectar Café. I have been approached to stock my products at some of the biggest and most incredible stores. Every time I have to turn down an opportunity it makes me feel like a failure, useless . . . all that stuff comes up. But then I think why I'm making that decision. My priorities right now are: kids first, business second.
>
> 'When I expand the business, I will have to give up so much of what is important to me. This is the choice I'm making, right now. I'm sure you're having to make one, too.'

LIFE ISN'T PERFECT?
DO SOMETHING FOR SOMEONE ELSE

One way to learn to be grateful for what you have is to help others. There are so many things you can do, starting with giving money or time to charities. But helping others doesn't just mean doing charity work, it can be doing any small thing for anyone who needs support.

In the yogic tradition, the service of helping others is called Seva, which means work performed without thought of reward or payment. Right now, as budgets are cut for essential community work, it's the ideal time to see what we can do within our own communities, how we can help someone who's having a harder time than we are.

Start with these small ways to be of service:

* Help someone with bags or a pram up some steps or onto a bus or tube. It takes one minute of your time and, as any mother with a pram will tell you, it's the best when someone offers help!

* Ask a homeless person if they want a coffee or a sandwich or a piece of cake. Maybe there's someone you see every day on your way to work?

* Donate to your local food bank. Or donate to a charity via direct debit, or support them by giving them your time or helping with a fundraiser. Shop in charity shops, too. Choose charities that have meaning to you, whether it's a women's charity or homeless shelter.

* Make an effort to say thank you – to everyone. It's always nice to know you've been noticed and acknowledged. In a relationship, after a while, it's easy to take your partner for granted, but remember how wonderful you thought your partner was when you met them?!

* Cook a meal and take it to someone who needs it, maybe an older neighbour, someone who's ill or grieving or just had a baby. Or just because you know someone is working hard and has little time to cook. We all know what a luxury it is to be fed a home-cooked meal when you're exhausted.

* Club together at work to help a particular cause that means something to you. There are loads of things you can do, from donating clothes to a women's shelter or organising a sports day to raise funds.

> Katia: 'When I was in my early 20s, living in LA, I used to volunteer in a hospice for people with AIDS. I'd go twice a week and do reiki on the patients. Every week I'd meet new patients and, over time, our relationships would develop. This was a time when AIDS was new and scary to most people, so to have someone come and touch the patients and support them going through the last months of their lives was a gift for them, but it was also a gift for me. At the time, I wasn't sure where my life was going, but every time I went there, knowing I was doing something that helped someone else, it made me feel good knowing I was of service in the world.'

CHANGE IS
GONNA COME

'You can't always choose what happens to you, but you can always choose how you feel about it.' *Danielle LaPorte*

Like it or not, your life is always changing, and so is everyone else's. What you need is the flexibility to roll with it. Think of a crop of wheat that is rooted and grounded but still able to bend in the wind. If you're unable to roll with it, change will inevitably feel both frightening and exhausting. Are you able to be flexible or are you so rigid that you freak out when things don't go to plan?

Nadia talks about this when she's teaching yoga, because yoga isn't just about learning to touch your toes, but about the ability to be flexible and graceful and light in all areas of your life.

There's good change, the things we plan and hope for, then there are unexpected changes. Some of Nadia's yoga pregnancy class students tell her after they give birth, 'No one ever told me it was going to be this lonely or hard.' There is no 'me' in those first months, it's all about the baby.

Maybe your change is the actual Change, the menopause, or perhaps you're building a business, trying to buy a flat, leaving a relationship, splitting up a business relationship or leaving the safety of a regular income to do something you believe in. These are all changes that can leave us questioning ourselves.

Other people change, too; it can be hard to accept that a friend is now in a different place in her life to where you are.

It's easy to freak out about change. If change scares you, maybe you deal with the difficulty by drinking alcohol or eating too much or too little, or just plain freezing and giving up control so you don't have to take responsibility.

When change feels overwhelming, our routines tend to fall apart, but this is when you need them the most. See where you can ground yourself. This will give you the stability that allows you to be more flexible elsewhere in your life. Root yourself firmly by prioritising sleep and exercise, and eating well. Those things may seem simple and obvious, but they will give you space while things feel unsettled.

> Nadia: 'I resisted buying a flat for years, until I realised it wasn't because I was the happy-go-lucky, it-is-what-it-is, carefree person I imagined. I realised it was because I was, frankly, terrified of financial commitment. I had to go through my fear of change, of becoming tied down, to get to what I really needed and always wanted – a home. The funny thing was, I was so scared of the idea of being "tied down" and stuck but now I rarely want to leave my flat because I love it so much!'

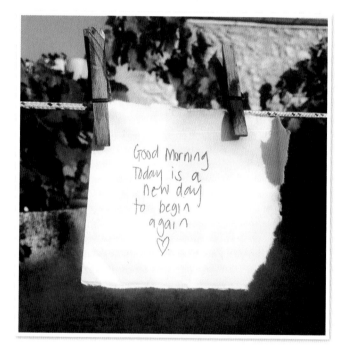

REMIND YOURSELF WHAT
YOU CAN DO

* Hardly anyone is good at looking back and seeing what they've accomplished. Write a list of what you have achieved so far in life, especially if it was against the odds.

* Even if you don't have the conventional outward signs of success – a house, a loving partner, picture-perfect children – you will have achieved incredible things. Focus on the fact that while other people's changes might be obvious and external, yours may be internal.

* Think about other times when you've made it through. You're reading this book, so you've made it this far. As Gloria Steinem, who is still rocking it in her eighties, says, 'The good thing about being old; you've seen when things have been worse.'

* Write down a time when you nailed a super-difficult challenge. How did you feel before, during and after your moment of victory? Next time you're challenged, think of that time and remember, you've got this, too.

WHEN YOU HAVE TO MAKE
A BIG DECISION

There are crossroad moments in everyone's life where, whatever you decide, it feels as if it will impact your life forever. You may be feeling the pressure of a big decision; maybe taking a new job, or deciding whether to split up with your partner or change an aspect of your life you're not happy with. Your friends may give you good advice, but ultimately no one can tell you for sure what will happen. All you can do is make a decision with your gut and the information that you have in the moment.

Even if, later, you wish you'd made a different decision, be kind to yourself and remember that you made the best decision you could with the information you had at the time. Don't beat yourself up for the things you didn't know back then.

So how can you know what the right thing to do is right now?

* Get a little bit of quiet and listen to yourself. You will have the answer, although it's not always easy to hear.

* Ask other people – but don't necessarily follow their advice. Sometimes friends who love you say what they know you want to hear. Or, with the best intentions, they give you suggestions based on their experiences, not yours. You need to make the right decision for you. You are the one who will have to live with it.

* Ask yourself: would it be bad to stay the same and not make the decision at all? What would happen if you did nothing?

* Make a list of pros and cons. Keep writing until your course of action becomes clear.

* Think about what you would regret, for each of your options.

* Get a professional opinion from a therapist or life coach. An outside person with no vested interest can have a perspective that you and your loved ones might not.

> Katia: 'A good friend, at the age of 38, was in love with a man who didn't want children, when she did. She had to decide what was more important to her: a child or the relationship. I said, "You have to decide what you need and want. The worst thing would be to stay with him, but blame him for not having a family. Even if you split up with him, and end up not having a child, at least you will have made the decision based on what you needed and wanted in that moment."'

NOTICING THOUGHTS MEDITATION

In Buddhism it's said that the one thing that's always guaranteed is life changes. The whole practice of meditation is about learning to sit and observe whatever is happening without attaching judgement to it. This teaches you to observe change without getting caught up in a story line where you project into the past or the future.

Sit still and concentrate on your breath. You don't have to cross your legs or sit in a lotus pose (unless you want to), just sitting in a chair is fine.

You'll notice your thoughts changing constantly, maybe from 'I'm so happy everything is great' to 'I'm such an asshole, why did I say that?' Just observe your thoughts and how they keep changing. Let the thoughts happen, and try not to get caught up in them.

Accept the changing nature of your thoughts and keep coming back to your breath; let your breath be your anchor.

NATURE CURE

Walking in nature, whether in a city park or out in the countryside, is a great practice for your whole being. It helps you appreciate change, especially unwanted change, if you're going through a rough time.

Choose a place near enough that you can take that walk every day, or at least weekly.

Take the same path each time you walk, really looking and noticing everything that surrounds you. You'll see tiny signs of change everywhere, from walk to walk. In winter, the trees are bare and the earth is covered with dead leaves. Then come the snowdrops and the first buds of spring. A few weeks later bluebells and other flowers appear, and the grass springs to life. As summer comes, plants grow tall and everything seems to bloom at once, then in the autumn you'll see fruits ripen, leaves drop and mushrooms appear.

When you really notice all of these changes around you, instead of stomping past lost in your own internal thoughts, or rushing by, or missing it because you are plugged into headphones, you'll start to feel part of the natural cycle of life. Then instead of panicking at the idea of change, or wanting to run away, you'll slowly become a little more at ease with it.

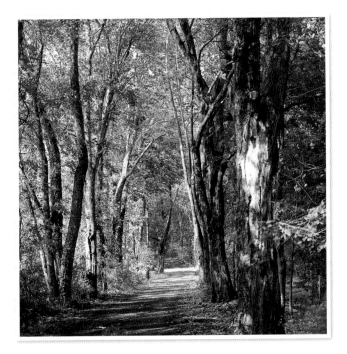

BREAK IT DOWN

When it all feels too much and you can't see a way forward, just stay close to what needs to be done right now. Think in little steps, not huge leaps. Break it down, make a plan. Ask yourself: what do I need to do today? Then make today's list. If you try to think ahead to everything you need to do, you'll crack.

* State your aim or goal. Perhaps you need to clear out the house of someone you love who has died, or maybe you have a happy goal, like planning a wedding.

* Let go of other stuff in your life that doesn't support the goal you're working towards right now. Make space for that goal.

* Work out what resources you need to achieve your goal. Is there anyone who can help you? Is there a trusted person who can advise you? Create a list or even a mood board to figure out exactly what you want.

* Make a list of what to do, when. Work out when things need to happen and put the timings in your diary. Make more lists! Prioritise what needs your attention first. Don't overwhelm yourself, take it in baby steps.

* Start working through one thing at a time by giving yourself a few hours a day when your goal has your full attention. Make sure it doesn't consume you, and that you have down time to refuel yourself.

* Remember that everything will come together in the end . . . then you can congratulate yourself. (Or get yourself a wedding planner!)

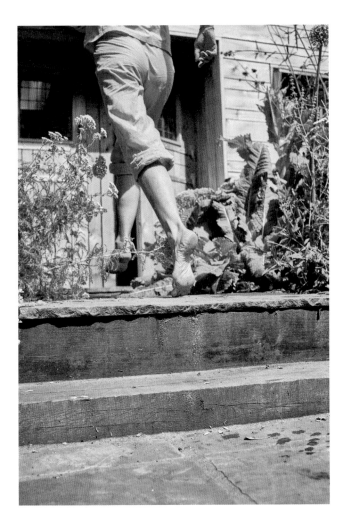

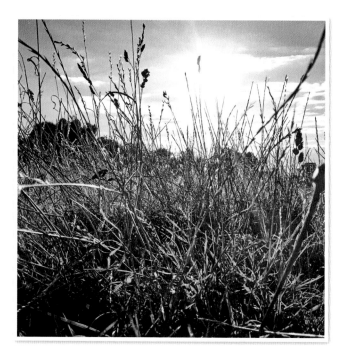

HOW TO BRING
MORE HOPE
INTO YOUR LIFE

* Check in with yourself. Notice how you feel. Do this every day, a few times a day if you can.

* Ask yourself, what does hope feel like to you? What do you feel hopeful about right now?

* When do you feel you are not aligned with the feeling of hope? What makes you feel worried or anxious, and what can you do about that?

* Ask yourself, what would hopefulness feel like right now in this moment?

* What could you do, right now, to feel more hope in your life?

* Do something for yourself today that brings you hope.

peace

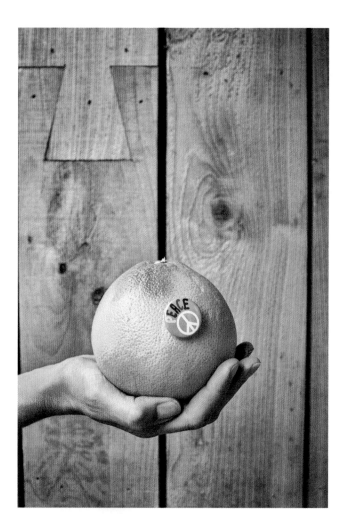

'Let what comes, come. Let what goes, go. Find out what remains.' Ramana Maharshi

When was the last time you felt peaceful? For a lot of us, it's hard to pinpoint that moment because feeling a sense of peace, ease and balance may be so unfamiliar that we struggle to remember it.

It is also because peace is the opposite feeling to stress, which is something we're all much more familiar with. Being busy and stressed can feel normal to us, but when we cultivate peace and approach life from that place, we're able to respond to the world in a more intelligent, thoughtful way than when we're running from commitment to commitment.

You might look at some of the headings in this section of the book and think, wait – heartbreak, grief, illness – these things aren't peaceful! We admit these aren't peaceful times in anyone's life, but that is exactly when you need peace, calm and balance the most. When life doesn't feel okay, just a moment of peace can help you feel that everything might be okay at some point in the future. We're not saying just have a quiet few minutes and all of your problems will go away, what we're saying is, at times of great personal strain, make sure you do small, good things for yourself every day.

Be gentle with yourself, as if you were looking after a friend who's going through tough times. You wouldn't tell her to pull herself together and get on with things. You'd be kind and considerate of her fragile state. Find some moments away from the onslaught of life and emotions, and that will leave you stronger and better able to get through them.

WHEN YOU'RE STRESSED

'The truth will set you free, but first it will piss you off.' *Gloria Steinem*

'How are you?' 'Oh, you know, busy.' Is that your usual answer? Being constantly busy can feel like a badge of honour, indicating to others that your life is full, you've people to see, places to go . . . It's a signal to the rest of the world that you're not lonely, or needy. Being busy tells everyone you're wanted; your time is precious and in demand.

Why not try to make some of that time precious for you? If you don't leave any gaps in your life for your body and mind to process the ridiculousness that is the fast pace of modern life, the stress builds up.

Some people feel the need to fill every moment of the day with activity. Or they feel guilty when they're not doing something or worrying about doing something.

Self-care reminds you that you need time being, not doing.

If you're feeling stressed, are shouting at people or getting ill, these are signs that you need more gaps in your life. These gaps are whatever self-care practice works best for you – it could be yoga, cooking, exercise, lying still, or even just pottering around with nothing important to do. When was the last time you didn't have to be anywhere? When every moment feels accounted for, it's hard not to feel like it's all getting on top of you.

You could get up ten minutes early and use that time to just sit and be, maybe make yourself a cup of tea and drink it in silence. Or you can do some meditation to clear your mind – the sense of peace it gives you will help you throughout the day.

How do you know what makes a good gap for you? It's how it makes you feel afterwards, for the rest of the day, for the next day and even beyond.

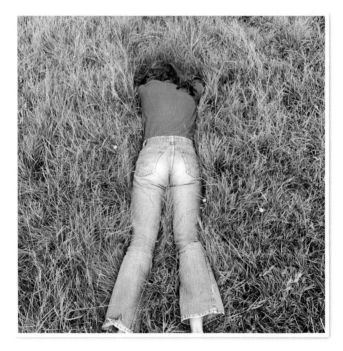

IN SEARCH OF THE
WORK/LIFE BALANCE

Do you look at other people's lives and think they have it all sorted? They're probably looking at yours and feeling the same. But we don't believe that anyone has it absolutely together all the time.

Work/life balance is great when it happens – but life always gets in the way. Most of us are just doing our best, going from one thing to the next. It can help to think of work/life balance as something that is achieved over the space of a month, or a year, rather than day to day.

There will always be days when you have to prioritise family over work, or vice versa. If you have children, run a business, have dependent relatives or friends, deadlines to meet, a job, or any kind of responsibilities, you have to accept that things will go wrong from time to time. All you can do in that moment of crisis, however big or small, is try to fix the things you can and surrender to the things you can't – and take care of yourself. It is better for you to embrace and accept the mess for what it is, instead of fighting against it.

When the immediate panic is over, this might be a great time to figure out where you can make some space for yourself to get perspective – maybe take a walk, or do some meditation or exercise that clears your head.

Even though we accept that the work/life balance is elusive, we believe you can still put systems in place to take some of the pressure off yourself. Just like the self-care savings in your bank, having some of these systems established as a habit will act as a buffer for times when everything goes crazy.

* Be more organised than you ever thought possible. Put everything you need to do in a diary and/or planner and your phone. Put alarms on your phone for daily and weekly tasks, and anything else that comes up. Enlist the other people in your household by having regular diary catch-ups. Empower children (and your partner) to be in charge of their own PE kit/homework schedule/club schedule.

* Practise setting boundaries. You need to be able to say no to anything that adds to your to-do-list burden without giving you something back. We're not saying don't help out your loved ones, but don't help out to the extent that your own life falls apart. Make a list of the things in the past month that you could have said no to; making cakes for school, organising a work lunch, an evening out with a friend you felt obligated to. If these things come up again, say no.

* Make time to do the things you love. It's always personal time that's the first thing to get knocked off the to-do list. What is the thing you love to do most? And when did you last do it? Put that at the top of the list, and underline it.

* Turn your phone off at least once a day. Create your own silent sanctuary where nobody can get to you. Try switching off your phone in the evenings. You don't need to have instant access to other people, or them to you all the time. We remember having to write letters to communicate with people (and it wasn't that long ago!)

* Clear your mind so you're not thinking of what you've got to do all the time. Making lists helps here, but so does having time to yourself out of your day. Meditation is the absolute best tool for this – if you really can't meditate, try active relaxation (see next page).

IF YOU CAN'T SLOW DOWN, PRACTISE ACTIVE RELAXATION

If meditation makes you anxious and the thought of sitting seems impossible, your self-care doesn't have to be about sitting still. Sometimes you need to move to feel better; to get out of your head and into your body. Nadia likes to do yoga for this, Katia likes to cook, but you can find your own way to calm your mind and look after yourself. Put it in your diary, like an appointment with yourself, so that it gets done.

* Practise yoga. It gives you a connection to your body, helps to still the mind and gives a feeling of connection. It teaches you to be aware of your breath as you move, which helps to calm your whole system.

* Choose some of your favourite songs and get dancing! One song usually lasts only three to four minutes, so you can time exactly how long you spend doing this. Moving to music that lifts your mood helps you feel joy and gives you a natural high.

* Cook something. If you choose a new or slightly complicated recipe you will have to pay proper attention, which makes you clear your mind of other thoughts without having to try to be mindful. The creativity of cooking and the pleasure of feeding others can be uplifting, too.

* Walk or run in the park or outdoors. Not only is being surrounded by green space known to lift your mood, running is also a great way to boost feel-good hormones.

* Write in a journal. If you write things down as they're happening, it gets them out of your system and onto paper. It's good to look at later, too, when things have moved on, to see how well you've dealt with situations and gone beyond them. It's also another good reminder that the bad feelings don't stick around.

CHECK YOURSELF

Your body starts giving you signs when you're doing too much, so pay attention to them. Maybe you feel run down, or get ill, or just feel a little overwhelmed. Learn to listen to your body's early warning system and see if you can take some time to rest and recuperate before you get worse. For some people, the first sign of stress is a headache, for others it's fatigue or feeling emotional.

You may have got used to being busy, but let your body answer the question 'Is this working for you?' If it isn't, what can you do that resources you, rather than depletes you?

It's useful to check in with your stress levels regularly, rather than just keep on keeping on, so you can tweak your days accordingly. Checking in and slowing down will stop daily stress turning into mind and body stress. When you check in, think about these questions:

* Am I getting any joy in life? When was the last time I laughed?

* Is the feeling of being overwhelmed always too much? Or is it sometimes a bit exciting and enjoyable?

* Is my glass half empty or full to the brim – or is it at least more full than empty?

* How do I feel physically? You could be getting neck or back pains, digestion issues or headaches; you know your personal signs.

* Am I doing too much? If so, how could I do less?

PUT YOURSELF IN YOUR OWN DIARY

Examine your diary looking both forwards and backwards. Go through each day. How did you spend each hour last week? Remember how you felt. Notice what didn't feel good to you.

* When you look at the week ahead, are you dreading any task, person, event or job in particular? What can you take out next week? Can you put in any time to relax or enjoy yourself? If there's nothing to cancel this week, is there anything next week? Is there anything you could give up long term?

* If you can't find anything to give up, highlight the chunk of time you usually spend zoning out on social media, watching box sets or worrying about other people.

* For a lot of people, the day runs away from them first thing, when they dive into emails or social media. Can you create a new, disciplined morning routine that feeds your mind and body? Maybe make a cup of tea and read something positive or inspirational. Then meditate or do yoga, even if it's only for ten minutes. It may mean getting up earlier (and going to bed earlier) but it will transform your whole day.

* Do you need to cut out a few nights out? Going out late a few nights in a row and drinking may feel fun in the moment, but it ain't going to feel fun in the morning. Do that night what you'll wish you'd done the next morning: be productive; read a book or watch a documentary, go to a yoga or fitness class, meditate, cook. Do something that feeds you rather than depletes you.

* Can you book a mental health day off work? Don't tell anyone else you're not at work or wherever you're supposed to be. Do something different on that day, visit a gallery or museum, try a new walk or go to the cinema on your own. This can be hard to do when you're self-employed, but instead of feeling you've lost money for the day, look at it as an investment in your sanity, which will make you a happier person and better at your job. And it's only one day.

* If not a whole day, can you book a mental health hour? A friend who works from home has put a really cosy day bed into her spare room. When she can, during the day, she makes herself a cup of tea and takes her book and her dog up to the room, closes the door and enjoys an hour reading and napping. Heaven.

* Can you reorganise your working life? The joy of doing a day a week from home is that you can get loads of work done while you're also loading your washing machine.

WATERCRESS, PEAR AND FENNEL JUICE

Watercress brings a delicious peppery flavour to this juice. If it's too spicy for you, try substituting some of the watercress with spinach.

Makes 2

bunch of watercress (approx. 100g)

2 pears, cored

2 fennel bulbs, roughly chopped

small thumb-sized piece of root ginger (no need to peel)

Juice all the ingredients and give the liquid a stir to make sure they're all combined. It's always best to juice the watercress (or any soft green leaf) first, then the harder fruit or vegetables will push the leaves through the juicer.

Cold-pressing preserves the enzymes for up to 4 days, but if you're not using a cold-press juicer, drink this straight away.

GREEN BEAUTY

A beautiful green smoothie with a taste of the tropics.

Makes 1

200ml coconut water

1 frozen peeled banana

50g baby spinach

1 tsp coconut oil

1 tsp bee pollen (optional)

50g frozen mango chunks

juice of ¼ lime

Whiz all the ingredients in a blender until smooth. Add more water if it is too thick for you.

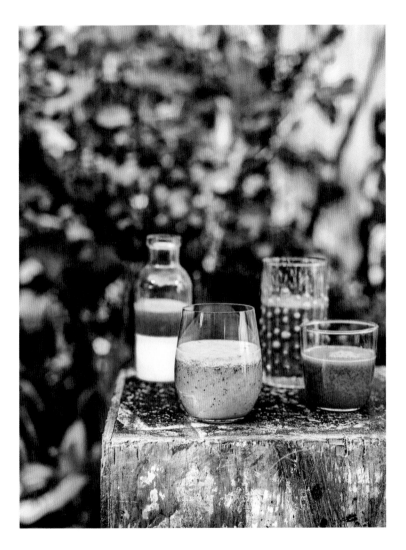

PINEAPPLE GRAPEFRUIT TURMERIC JUICE

This makes a gorgeous drink with a bright yellow colour from the turmeric. Be super careful with the raw turmeric as it will stain everything – this is not the time to wear your favourite white sweater!

Makes 2

¼–½ pineapple
(approx. 200ml
of juice)

1 large pink grapefruit
(approx. 200ml
of juice)

10 mint leaves

small thumb-sized
piece of root
ginger, unpeeled
(approx. 50g)

finger of turmeric
root, unpeeled
(approx. 20g)

Peel and chop the pineapple, then juice it. If using a cold-press juicer, peel and juice the grapefruit. If you have a centrifugal juicer, it's better to squeeze the grapefruit instead.

Next pass the mint, ginger and turmeric through the juicer and combine with the fruit juices.

COLD-BREW GREEN TEA

This is so easy and refreshing. Not only can you taste the delicate flavour of the green tea, but the cold-brew method releases less caffeine than using boiling water.

Make sure you use a good-quality loose-leaf green tea and, most importantly, good water – spring or filtered water is best.

1 tbsp green oolong tea leaves

1 litre water

Mix the tea leaves with the water in a jug and leave overnight in the fridge. The next day, strain out the leaves and discard them.

This cold-brew tea will last a week in the fridge, as long as you've strained out the leaves first.

ASK FOR HELP

It can often be easier to help others than to ask for or accept help ourselves. People sometimes think needing help makes them look weak or vulnerable, or they feel ashamed they can't do it all on their own. Remember, though, no one can do everything on their own all the time. Asking for help is a sign of strength, and once you've been helped, you can pay it back by helping someone else.

* Consider therapy: if you can't get it free (ask your GP) it might be the best money you spend. You don't have to have a specific problem; therapy can do deep things such as enable you to work out your whole being, but it can also do more everyday things, such as help you handle difficult conversations, support you if you're feeling unsure, negative or insecure. We all have that friend who's got stuck, repeating the same negative pattern over and over – or is that you? At some point you will have to get help for it.

* If you feel you've got too much on and you're going around saying 'I'm about to have a nervous breakdown', let people help you, but respect their boundaries and make sure this is a short-term thing, not a habit.

* Ask a friend if you can come over for dinner.

* Ask other school parents if they can pick up your kids from school.

* Call your sibling and ask if they can go and visit your mother/father this week, if you can't.

* Put in a request with your boss for some back-up on a certain piece of work.

* See if a colleague or professional mentor can help you with a problem or with contacts.

Don't forget to thank the people who've helped you. Give flowers or a handwritten note to let your friends know their kindness was appreciated. Don't take people's help for granted; it may have cost them a lot – in terms of time if not money. And always offer to return a favour.

A TRICK FOR INSTANT CALM

This may sound absolutely bizarre, but try it.

When Katia was doing back-to-back massages on clients, it got pretty tiring. So, when she had a break, she'd lie down on the massage table and imagine herself being massaged. Crazy as it sounds, it helped her to feel relaxed and regenerated for the next client. It's now a technique we both use when we're on the go – though we'd prefer a hands-on massage any day!

Nuts, right? But worth a shot.

GETTING PROACTIVE ABOUT
SELF-CARE

* Have a massage. Being touched physically helps release the stress from your body. Treat yourself at least every couple of months, if you can. Or try the self-massage on page 30.

* Breathing release. Lie down on your back and place one hand palm-down on your heart, the other palm-down on your belly. As you breathe in and out through your nose, scan your body to feel where you have tension or discomfort. Rub your palms together until they're warm, then put your hands in that place. If the pain is emotional, put your hands on your heart. If it's mental, put your hands on your head. Take five deep breaths.

* Back release. Tension, for most of us, ends up in the back. This technique is an excellent release. Take two towels and roll them up together vertically to make one long roll. Lie down on the roll so it presses along the length of your spine. Spread your arms and legs out in a star shape, relax everything, and lie still for five to ten minutes, breathing deeply with your eyes closed.

* Legs up the wall. Lie on your bed with your bum against the headboard or wall, then lift your legs so they are resting on the wall with the soles of your feet facing the ceiling. Lie in that position for five to ten minutes. This helps to relax tired leg muscles, quiet the mind and calm the nervous system. It's great to do just before bed.

* Relaxing body scan. Sit or lie down and first bring your attention to your breathing. Then start to notice the whole of your body and where you may be holding, gripping or contracting any parts of yourself – and let them go. Start at your feet and work all the way up your body to your head, going through each part of the body and relaxing it. Take your time, taking a few breaths at each point. Think these words to yourself for each body part: I

relax my feet. I relax my legs. I relax my buttocks. I relax my back. I relax my hands and arms. I relax my belly. As I breathe in my belly rises, as I breathe out it softens. I let my head feel heavy and relaxed. I let my eyes relax, my lips and jaw soften and relax. I let my whole body feel heavy and relaxed. Every part of me is relaxing.

* Tennis ball massage. If you sit at a desk on a chair with a back at work, this is a great one to do. It's also really good to take your tennis ball on the plane when you travel, too, so that you can do this on long flights.

   Place a tennis ball between your back and your chair and lean back into it. Find the tight spots around your shoulders or shoulder blades, then wiggle around on the ball and feel those tight spots loosen. You can do this lying on the floor, too, if you prefer.

* Jaw massage. Your jaw holds a lot of tension; this massage can help you release it. Make fists with your hands then, starting just underneath your earlobes and using a circular motion, work your knuckles around your jawline from your ears all the way to your chin.

* Take a walk. Earlier in the day is ideal if you live in the city, because it's easier to feel relaxed when there are fewer people around. Try to walk, most days, for 30 to 40 minutes at a time.

HEARTBREAK

Your heartbreak may be recent and you don't know what to do with yourself, except lie on the sofa listening to sad songs on repeat. If the heartbreak is older, you've gone on about it to friends and family, likely more than once and possibly after a few drinks. Maybe they've started to talk about online dating, saying it's time to move on, and you just want to scream.

Heartbreak comes in all shapes and sizes. Either way, it feels pretty shitty and you're sick of running to the loos to cry at inconvenient times. Then, if you don't seem to be feeling any better when everyone says you're 'meant to', you can start worrying about that, too.

First thing: stop beating yourself up about being sad. If you break your leg you're expected to take some time to heal, right? Nobody is going to expect you to run a marathon the next week. The cast protects the leg until the bone has healed. Then, and only then, are you expected to be able to have the plaster removed and show the world your skinny, pale, hairy leg! But we don't give heartbreak the same care or time that we give to a broken bone.

Friends and family are usually able to listen for the first few weeks, when you need to get it off your chest, but after a while you might feel you can't inflict it on them any more. Don't beat yourself up or feel like a loser for having feelings. Instead, you need to think of this as a time to put your heart in a plaster cast. There is something to be said for sitting with the sad emotions for an allocated, specific period of time, and really feeling them. That doesn't mean you won't feel them again afterwards, of course you will, but you need to get right into that sadness and let it move through you, rather than pretend it's not there and keep it stuck inside.

The time it will take to heal isn't predictable and doesn't always reflect the importance of the relationship; sometimes a super-long, healthy relationship can take hardly any time to get over compared to a short fling with someone who rejected you, which can feel like forever. This is fine, too, just let yourself feel the way you feel.

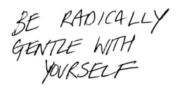

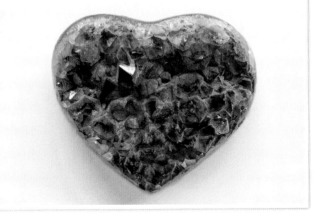

HOW TO FEEL THE FEELINGS

A break-up can throw up a hard-to-swallow mix of complicated emotions.

There's grief and also sadness over the loss of the partnership or family you might have imagined for your future. He or she might have been the person you wanted to have children with and now you're scared you may never have them. There's also hope: might you get back together? At some point you'll feel angry: how could they be such a dick? Oh, and there might be shame; perhaps you think you weren't good enough for them because of some fault you find with yourself.

Self-care means feeling the feelings and letting them pass through you. If you pretend they're not happening, or try to change how you feel, or pull yourself together before you're ready, it will take longer to get over it. You might think you need to get out there, and your friends might be saying that too, and you may get out there and then find it feels worse! It only heals when it heals, and you will be done when you are done.

Scientists have shown that rejection uses the same pathway in the brain as physical pain, and triggers the same chemicals in your brain as withdrawal from addiction. So, no, you're not imagining the pain. People who have been rejected can take it much harder than if a relationship simply didn't work out. Being rejected, even from a short relationship, can leave you feeling as if you're going a bit mad.

Watch out, though; there is a fine line between feeling your feelings and just drowning in them.

WHAT TO DO WHEN YOU'RE HEARTBROKEN

* When you're going through difficult times, do one nice thing for yourself every day. If you can manage just one lovely meal, a walk, five minutes to yourself, a call with a good friend, a massage, you're supporting yourself to get through it. Or go and find a yoga class, head to the gym or out for a run.

* After a friend finally broke up with a long-term partner she went to a spa for a whole day with her best friend. She treated herself to nearly every treatment and said she felt much better for it. Expensive, but effective, in her case.

* Try colouring. We would never have thought of this ourselves but a cousin told us this break-up story and it was brilliant. She chose a really beautiful colouring-in book after breaking up with her boyfriend, and she spent three months perfecting a single picture. She would sit side by side with her mum, both of them colouring and talking about things she needed to discuss. Now the picture is finished, it looks incredible; she has something to be proud of for that time and she's processed her feelings and moved on.

* Reboot your creativity. Artists and musicians always talk about the creativity that comes from heartbreak: maybe you can use your sadness as a burst of creative energy? Take a class and learn something new: pottery or writing. Concentrating and focusing your energy will take you out of your thoughts, and it's a good way of meeting new people and building your confidence.

* Buy some inspirational self-help books and see how you can grow from this experience.

WHAT <u>NOT</u> TO DO WHEN
YOU'RE HEARTBROKEN

* Don't stalk your ex on social media. You don't want to see them having a good time, whether they're on a night out with friends or, most especially, with what looks like their new love interest. In fact, why not swear off social media for a month? Even if you unfollow your ex, or block them, your mutual friends are going to tag them, and you'll still see them going about their life – albeit a positively edited life with just the good bits. You don't have to do this forever, just until you've healed a bit.

In the same vein, don't like your ex's pictures on Instagram, or tweet coded messages that are aimed at them, or try to create a story on social media that you've moved on. It's all a waste of energy and not real. Instead do some healing and spend time on yourself.

* Don't drink and dial. Or text. Or email. You're feeling alone, so you're reaching out to your ex to fill your emptiness. In the moment you can talk yourself into believing it's the right thing to do; it's definitely not. Good friends will stop you – listen to them! Delete all numbers and emails. Don't write letters to your ex telling them how great the relationship was and what they're missing out on.

* Don't plan a revenge evening. You're thinking, 'I'm going to go out and they're going to see me looking fabulous, and want me back.' It doesn't work like that. By all means look amazing, but do it to *feel* amazing, not for an ex.

* Don't sleep with your ex's friends. That's not revenge, that's you pressing your own self-destruct button.

* Don't talk about your ex with your friends incessantly. Of course you can talk about them, but don't make your ex the primary focus of your nights in or out.

* Don't blame yourself. Sometimes a break-up happens because of bad timing, it's nothing personal. Or maybe you have a lesson to learn about yourself. Remember that you were okay before you met your ex and you will be okay after they've gone. We create these stories about our lives: the perfection of what our life was like as a couple, your favourite pub or restaurant or walk, but the reality is you were going to those places before you were together and you will continue to do so.

> Nadia: 'Once, after a break-up, I was walking through a farmers' market reminiscing about how I missed doing the Sunday shop with my ex. Then I remembered I'd never gone with him to the farmers' market in the first place! Sometimes the fantasy can be bigger than reality.'

TRY TIE-CUTTING

No, we don't mean going into his wardrobe and cutting his ties with scissors. This ritual, energetic tie-cutting is about symbolically cutting the emotional ties you have with an ex, so you can get on with your life without them. It does sound a bit weird and witchy, but it's not harmful – and it's very simple.

Some people get scared about doing this, worried that the person will have nothing to do with them afterwards, but while it might turn out like that, the result could also be that the relationship will take its form in a healthier way, maybe as a friendship.

This ritual needs to be done with kindness, not with hate or anger. Sitting somewhere peaceful, say out loud: 'Whatever belongs to me, I return to me. And whatever is yours I return to you. I send you away with love.' See threads connecting the two of you and imagine gently cutting them away.

That's it.

SWEET POTATO FRITTERS
WITH YOGURT PAPRIKA SAUCE

*I love these, my kids love these, and when I make them
for other people I always make an extra batch for myself!
When you fry the patties the corn goes all charred and
delicious – my favourite bit. This makes a lot but you can
freeze the patties in a plastic Tupperware box, in layers
separated with baking parchment. Allow them to defrost
at room temperature, then just reheat them in the oven
for 10–15 minutes.*

**Makes about
12 fritters**

*1 sweet potato,
about 400g*

*bunch of spring onions
(approx. 100g),
finely chopped*

*1 red chilli, deseeded
and finely chopped*

*3 tbsp olive oil (maybe
a little more)*

200g kale, leaves only

*1 x 340g tin sweetcorn,
drained*

100g ground almonds

½ tsp salt

zest of 1 lemon

2 eggs

*3 tbsp plain flour
(you can use any
alternative flour here,
the idea is just to
bind the ingredients)*

Preheat the oven to 190°C/360°F/Gas mark 5.

Wash the sweet potato and poke a few holes in it with
a skewer or a knife so that it cooks all the way through.
Bake in the oven for about 1 hour until the sugars start
to run out of the skin and caramelise.

Meanwhile, sauté the spring onions and chilli in
1 tablespoon of olive oil over a low heat until soft.

Blanch the kale leaves in boiling water for 1 minute,
then drain and leave to cool before squeezing the
water out. In a large mixing bowl, combine the kale,
corn, spring onions, chilli, ground almonds, salt and
lemon zest.

Once the sweet potato is done, scoop out the golden
sweetness, mash it and add to the mixture in the bowl.
In a small bowl, beat the eggs and add to the rest of
the ingredients with the flour. Combine everything with
your hands and scoop about 2 tablespoons of mix out
per fritter. Flatten these into little patties and set aside.

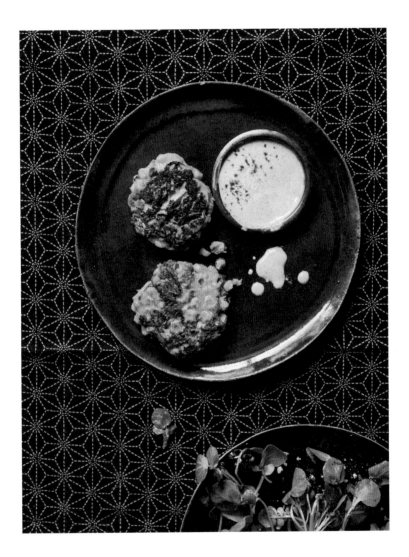

For the yogurt
  paprika sauce
75g plain yogurt
¼ tsp smoked paprika
juice of ½ lemon
pinch of salt

Combine all the yogurt sauce ingredients.

Heat the remaining olive oil in a large frying pan. Fry the patties in batches, over a medium heat, for about 4 minutes on each side until they're golden. Be careful as you flip them, they're delicate!

You'll need to wipe down the pan between batches with a piece of kitchen paper, and add more oil as you go along.

Serve three patties per person with the yogurt paprika sauce on the side and perhaps a green salad.

SPINACH AND PEA SOUP WITH TRUFFLE OIL

This is my Auntie Max's soup, which she makes every Friday night. I've added truffle oil to her recipe because I find it adds a delicious earthiness. I admit truffle oil is a luxury ingredient, but a little goes a really long way, and it's great to have in the cupboard. Try using leftover oil in scrambled eggs; it's also delicious with roasted pumpkin or drizzled over pasta with a grating of Parmesan.

Serves 5

2 tbsp olive oil
1 medium leek, chopped
200g spinach leaves
300g peas (frozen are fine)
750ml vegetable stock
½ tsp salt
pinch of black pepper
2½ tsp truffle oil

Heat the olive oil in a large saucepan on a low heat and add the chopped leek. Sauté until soft and sweet, which will take around 8 minutes.

Throw in the spinach and let the leaves wilt, then add the peas, stock, salt and pepper. Bring to a boil and let it all simmer for 5 minutes.

Take the pan off the heat to blend. If you're using a stick blender, you can just blend the soup in the pan, otherwise you'll need to let the soup cool a bit before you put it into the blender.

Once blended until smooth, divide the soup among five bowls and drizzle each with a little truffle oil – I use no more than half a teaspoon per serving, but adjust it to your own taste.

BUDDHA BOWLS

Buddha bowls are one of the most popular items on our café menu. They're an adaptation of the traditional monks' alms bowl; Buddhist monks go house to house to receive donations of food called the Pindapata – which means 'dropping a lump'.

To create your own bowl, we suggest starting with a grain or a noodle in the middle of the bowl, then arrange three or four other elements around the edge. Any more than that might be overwhelming.

It's good to try to have a sea vegetable or something fermented in your bowl, and lots of vegetables. Think about the colours of your bowl; you want it to be bright – too much of one colour will look bland. It doesn't have to be vegetarian, you can make these bowls with a really nice piece of fish.

I like to prepare the salads or pâtés at the weekend so I have all the makings of a bowl in the fridge for the week ahead. Add the avocado just before eating.

Makes 4 bowls

200g quinoa, cooked and cooled

4 tbsp wild green dressing (see page 50)

1 avocado

1 jar of raw fermented cabbage (sauerkraut)

4 tbsp beetroot pâté (see page 178)

60g toasted pumpkin seeds

Kale Salad

1 bag kale leaves (290g), finely chopped

Mix the cooked quinoa with the wild green dressing.

Combine the kale dressing ingredients in a bowl, and add to the kale. Massage with your hands until the kale becomes soft and glossy.

Next, combine the ingredients for the Carrot and Beetroot dressing in a bowl, and add to the grated carrots and beetroot.

Finally, cut the avocado in half then into quarters, and remove the skin by peeling it back neatly. Slice each

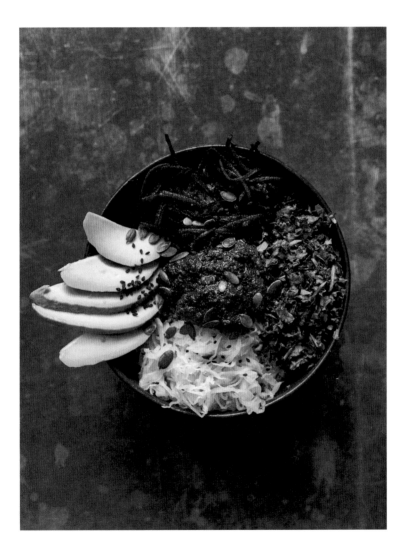

For dressing 1
2 tsp tamari
1 tbsp sesame oil
1 tsp rice vinegar
juice of 1 lime

Carrot and
  Beetroot Salad
1 raw beetroot, peeled
  and grated
2 large carrots, peeled
  and grated

For dressing 2
juice of 1 orange
50ml olive oil
75ml red wine vinegar
¼ tsp salt
¼ tsp black pepper

quarter of avocado into three at an angle.

Now assemble the bowls. Divide the quinoa among four bowls – this will be the centre of each bowl. Around this add equal portions of the carrot and kale salads. Add a similar amount of fermented cabbage. Arrange the avocado slices on the side of the bowl.

Put 1 tablespoon of beetroot pâté in the middle of each bowl, and top with a sprinkle of toasted pumpkin seeds to serve.

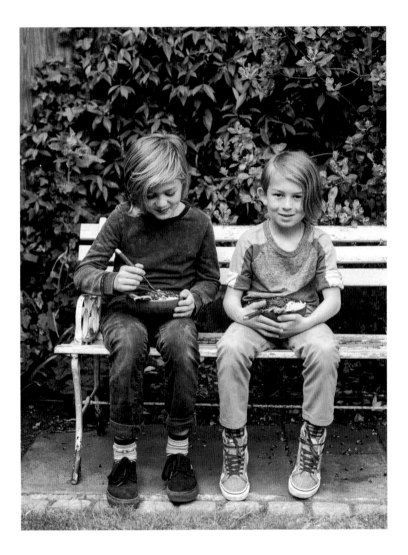

ROSE CHIA OVERNIGHT OATS

I was inspired to make this by one of my favourite chefs, Sabrina Ghayour. In her book Persiana she makes a rice pudding with rose water and cardamom, and I wanted to use those flavours to turn overnight oats into something really special. It's a great one to make at the weekend, and then you have breakfast sorted for the busy days ahead.

Makes 3

130g oats

2 tbsp chia seeds

330ml oat milk (or milk of your choice)

2 tsp runny honey

pinch of salt

pinch of ground cinnamon

1 tsp vanilla extract

zest of 1 lime

seeds from 2 cardamom pods, ground (or a pinch of ready-ground)

½ tsp rose water

Topping suggestions

chopped pistachios, pumpkin seeds or toasted almonds

dried rose petals

Mix the oats and chia seeds together in a bowl, then pour in the oat milk and really mix well so that there are no lumps of chia. Add all the remaining ingredients and stir to combine.

Cover the bowl and place in the fridge overnight. The next morning the oats will be thick and rich.

Just before eating, top with a small handful of chopped pistachios, pumpkin seeds, toasted almonds and a sprinkle of rose petals.

Overnight oats will keep in the fridge for up to 4 days.

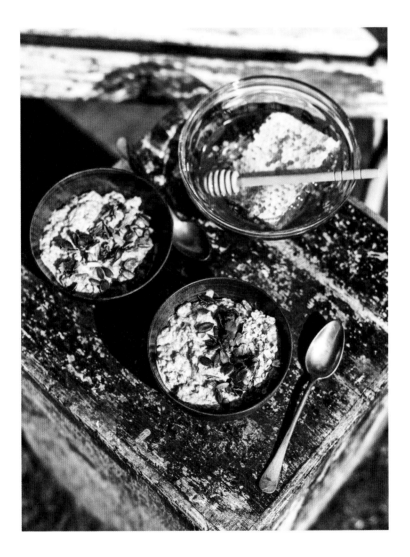

LOSING THOSE
YOU LOVE

'Know that one day your pain will become your cure.' *Rumi*

There's no silver lining to losing a person you love. It's going to be a painful time and there is no escape from it. You can't know how grief will affect you until you experience it – emotions can hit you unexpectedly, just when you thought you were doing fine. What you have to do is make the space for those feelings. Once you accept that, things may become a little easier to manage.

Allow yourself to be vulnerable, allow yourself to ask for help. We hope you have friends and family around you to help you. It can be hard to feel what you need to feel because you've got to behave a certain way at work, or you don't want to break down in front of other grieving people, or you have to hold it together in front of children.

* A bereavement counsellor may be the best investment of time, and money, that you can make at this moment. He or she will be trained to take you through the process of grieving. The goal is not that you get over someone, but that the loss becomes woven into the fabric of your life, instead of being the huge, gaping crater that it may seem right now.

* Find a support group of people you can talk to who have also lost a partner or loved one. Grief needs outside support. Bereavement feels devastating, but other people can resource you and ground you so you can deal with things better.

* Know everyone's reaction to grief is different. You don't know how grief is going to hit you so just be kind to yourself, honour it and don't try to rush the process. When our dad died, we dealt with it in completely different ways.

Katia: 'A few weeks after our dad died, I woke one night, sat bolt upright and had a huge, primal crying release. I didn't have the time or space to grieve any more, as I'd just found out I was pregnant.'

Nadia: 'When we had to organise Dad's stuff, and sort through what felt like his whole life, I hardly cried. But once I was back home, I cried uncontrollably at weird times. Sometimes I couldn't stop, which was really unlike me. That lasted for three months, almost daily.'

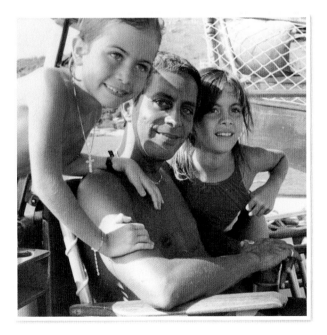

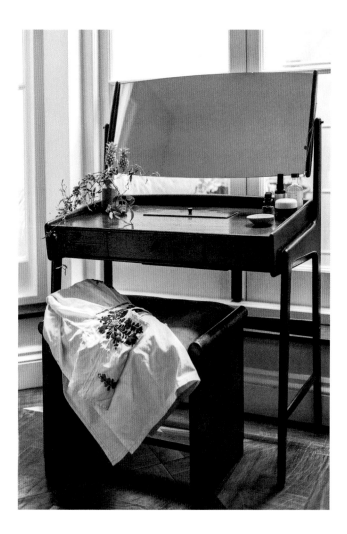

DO SOMETHING NICE FOR YOURSELF RIGHT NOW

There is no question that this is a time when you should do something nice for yourself every day. Our biggest message to you is: now is the time to step up your self-care. This is not the time to let things fall apart, even if you think you can't cope. You need to do at least one nice thing for yourself, every day, however small.

Once you've managed that, do one more.

When you're doing your nice thing for yourself, it's important to notice you're doing it. Consciously say to yourself, 'I'm going to do this thing for myself'. This sends a message that you are a priority.

BOOK IN FOR A
TOUCH THERAPY

When emotional pain is really bad, you may not want to talk about it, or you may not even be able to, so the emotions can get stuck in the body. That's why touch therapies like massage are worth prioritising during times of grief. As well as boosting your immune system, touch therapies help to alleviate stress, anxiety and depression.

Perhaps you're not convinced that emotions register in your body? But if you listen to your body, you might find you can feel your mind and body aren't separate. When something bad happens, it goes right to your stomach. When you get nervous, you may feel it on your chest or in your stomach, too. The whole of your body experiences your emotions.

In our society, we tend to ignore or push away feelings of anger or sadness. We think it's not right or appropriate or polite to express them. So they're left unprocessed. Children are brilliant because they can cry and have a tantrum, then they're over what was bothering them. It is important not to bypass the feelings we have even if they're not convenient or comfortable. It also helps to include the body when we're processing our feelings.

If you don't want to have a massage, could you get someone to give you a foot rub? Or get a manicure or a blowdry? You might feel that any of these ideas is a superficial indulgence when you're so deep in grief, but try it and you may be surprised how much it helps.

THINGS TO TRY WHEN
YOU'RE SAD

* Build an altar or shrine to the person you've lost. It may seem a little morbid, but it is simply a physical representation of how special that person is to you. You don't need to think of an altar as being religious, just find a surface where you can place pictures and objects that mean something to you or to the person you're mourning. When you're at the altar, talk to that person as if they were there, because your relationship continues, even if they've gone.

* Surround yourself with people who care. As grief can hit you at weird times you need to be around the right type of people. Those are the people who trust, know and love you, and who make you feel safe.

* Focus on getting quality sleep. Often people who are grieving find it hard to sleep, so make a sleep routine your priority (see page 252).

* Eat well. Make time to buy, cook and prepare fresh food or you'll risk getting more run down. Or let other people feed you.

* When people offer to help, take them up on it. You might feel as if nobody can do things the way you can, but let other people support you. Request that they do something specific: walk your dog, clean a room, sort your laundry, do a shop for you. Let other people look after you.

WHEN YOU'RE ILL

'Do not punish yourself for not always being at your best.'
Yung Pueblo

The idea of proper convalescence seems to have disappeared from modern life. But there's a lot to be said for the old-fashioned notion of rest and recuperation – simply staying in bed and resting, not pushing yourself to get back out there and pretending to be better.

Naturally your needs will depend on the illness you have, but whether it's a two-day cold or a condition you might have to live with for a long time, pushing yourself too hard, too early may not be the best thing to do.

When it comes to minor illnesses, we're not saying self-care will help you get better faster, but it might make being ill an easier experience. Cold and flu medicine adverts rely on the cultural assumption that we have got to power through our symptoms and get back to life quickly. But it's not skiving to wait until you're better before you go back to work.

Most of us seem to think if we can walk, we can work, but suppressing a cold with medication often seems to make it recur, and sometimes even turn into something worse. Nobody does their best work when they're ill; perhaps your body is telling you that what it needs, more than anything, is some time out.

So if you're not on top form, we're giving you permission to go back to bed – and stay there. Give yourself time to really heal and to rest. We hope you feel better soon.

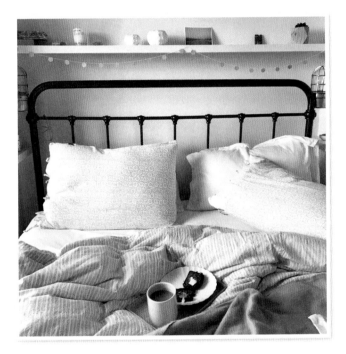

HOW TO CONVALESCE

(and how not to)

A couple of years ago, Katia went into hospital thinking she had appendicitis and ended up having a pretty major operation. It turned out she had a mass on her large intestine and she had to have a part of her ascending colon removed.

It was major. She was in hospital for a week and, even after that, it took three full months to return to her usual good health. When she was in hospital and convalescing at home afterwards, we paid a lot of attention to the things that felt good to her, and we realised what a difference self-care made to her mood and her recovery.

DO

* Put clean sheets on the bed. Ask someone to change your sheets every few days if you can. A clean bed is heaven when you're ill. If it's really impractical to change all the bedding, just change the bottom sheet and pillowcases, or even just the pillowcases.

* Make the bed comfortable with extra pillows for different sitting positions. Add a hot water bottle and an extra-soft blanket in winter, a light sheet instead of a duvet in summer.

* Put on clean nightwear. Lovely soft pyjamas, your favourite nightie, cosy bed socks, your softest old T-shirt, whatever feels right.

* Use aromatherapy oils and products. Good oils for illness are antibacterial tea tree oil, calming lavender and uplifting mandarin or orange.

Use your favourite oil in a diffuser to fragrance the room.

Put a few drops of lavender oil on your pillow or mix some drops of tea tree and lavender in a spray bottle with water and use as an air freshener instead of harsh chemical scents.

Placing a drop of food-grade peppermint oil on your tongue or inhaling a drop from your hands will lift your spirits and make you feel fresher.

* Take a daily bath or shower, if your illness allows. Or, if you've got a cough or cold and need to clear your airways, a twice-daily steam will get the phlegm moving.

* If you can move your body, try restorative yoga. It's good because it puts your system into the rest state, which helps your body recover from being over-stressed. If you can't move, try yoga nidra, a systematic deep-relaxation technique, which is more like meditation, in that you lie and listen to a soundtrack designed to relax your mind and body. There are hundreds of apps for yoga nidra, just find the one you like best.

* Sleep. Whenever you feel like it. Especially if you've been in hospital, which can be such a hard place to sleep, with the constant noise, lights and people. Then sleep some more.

* Treat yourself to some kind of physical touch, whether that is reflexology, head and neck massage or gentle body massage. This is especially beneficial if you have been in bed for long periods, as it helps with circulation and is great for your immune system.

* Ask for whatever help you need.

DON'T

* Keep watching box sets. It may feel luxurious to sit with your laptop or tablet in bed but it's not restful. While watching those shows, your mind is active and your nervous system is activated. It's proper rest that helps to restore you.

* Let too many visitors come. You don't want to see anybody who's going to tax you, be noisy, or ask anything of you. If this sounds like your children (it sounds like most children, to be honest), can you get someone else to look after them to allow you to rest? Only have visitors who are going to help you, not just people who feel they should come. And don't have too many people at once.

* Check in to work emails. You are ill – this can't be your responsibility right now. The people you work for will want you to get better, and you won't if you're taxing yourself. With important home and work issues, make sure someone else is responsible while you can't be.

A MEDITATION FOR HEALING

There is a simple but powerful self-healing meditation you can do whenever you feel the need. It is particularly effective if used when you feel the first symptoms of an illness, but it also works with illness that's entrenched if you do it at frequent intervals and with an intense focus.

We aren't suggesting a healing meditation is replacement for treatment from your doctor. But it can give you a mental and physical boost when illness has you feeling low.

When you are unoccupied for a few minutes, and especially last thing at night before falling asleep and first thing in the morning before getting up, 'flood' your body with healthy consciousness. This is how:

Lie flat on your back and close your eyes.

Relax your whole body and allow the ground beneath you to support you fully.

Focus on each organ of your body and imagine healing energy and light filling that organ. Give thanks to each organ in turn – your liver, your heart, your lungs, and so on – for all it does for you.

Fill your whole body, from your toes to the crown of your head, with the sensation of light and peace. Send gratitude and healing to the whole of your being.

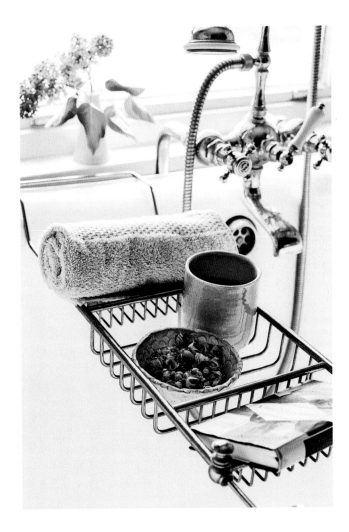

TAKE A HEALING BATH

Taking a restful bath is a great way to relax at the end of the day, and it all but guarantees a good night's sleep. You can turn a regular bath into a healing one with just a few simple additions. We're not claiming these baths can cure serious illness, but we hope they might make you feel a bit better in yourself. These are some of our favourites.

Bedtime bath. Epsom salts are super-rich in magnesium and wonderful for a bedtime bath, as they relax the muscles and get you ready for sleep. They don't need to be expensive – you can order a 5kg bag of Epsom salts online and keep them in a glass jar next to the bath, where they'll last for months. Use one cupful per bath.

Relaxing bath. Add three or four drops of relaxing lavender and chamomile essential oils to a tablespoon of milk in a jar. Put the lid on and give it a good shake before adding to a warm bath. Mixing with milk helps the oils disperse more evenly in your bath, rather than floating on the surface, but you can just add the oils directly to the water if you prefer.

Skin-calming bath. This is good for any inflammation, from eczema to insect bites and mild sunburn. Take a couple of handfuls of plain oats and either tie them up in a muslin square or put them in a sock and knot it. Tie the bundle to the tap and run the bath water through it. To calm irritated skin, add a drop of lavender oil.

A detoxing bath. Add one to two cups of apple cider vinegar to your bath. This is also good for clearing you energetically at the end of a hard day. Think of it as clearing your emotions as well as your physical body, if you've been around a lot of people or in difficult situations.

For sore muscles. Add five drops of rosemary essential oil and a cupful of Epsom salts.

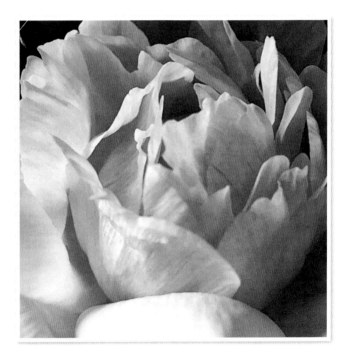

HOW TO FEEL
MORE PEACE

* Check in with yourself. Notice how you feel. Do this every day, a few times a day if you can.

* Ask yourself, what does peace feel like to you? Can you learn to feel it at times of stress, as well as at times of ease?

* When do you feel you are not aligned with the feeling of peace? What can you do to change that?

* Ask yourself, what would a sense of peace feel like right now in this moment?

* What could you do, right now, to feel more peace in your life?

* Do something for yourself today that brings you peace.

joy

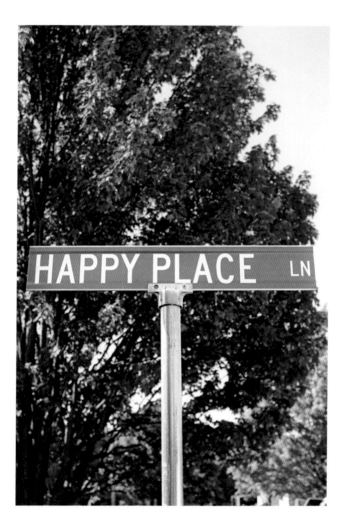

'Joy is the best make up.' *Anne Lamott*

True, lasting joy comes from making peace with who you are, and why you are here. You don't find joy in buying or acquiring or doing, but from being. Of course there is great joy to be found in your friends, family and relationships, but it's important to remember that true joy doesn't rely on external events, people or things.

We want to show you how to access your joy with self-care, by creating boundaries, seeing beyond any passing mood, however dark, and making sure you're not driving yourself too hard.

A sense of joy changes your perception of everything that happens to you. It affects how you behave and makes the world seem a better place.

Being connected to your inner joy can truly change your life.

SELF-CARE IN RELATIONSHIPS

'The world is full of nice people, if you can't find one, be one.' *Rumi*

The less good you feel about yourself, and the less joy you feel inside, the more likely you are to seek relationships with the wrong people. Instead of looking for a person who brings out the best in us, when we're feeling low we often seem to gravitate towards someone who mirrors how we feel inside.

When you tap into the feeling of joy that is always in you, you are more likely to attract someone who matches that vibration. Cultivating your own sense of joy allows you to be the best version of yourself in any relationship.

What does a good relationship mean to you? Is it being with someone who always has your back and you always have theirs? Someone who makes you laugh? We think the best relationships are those where your partner can tell you when you are not being the best version of yourself . . . and who can love you even then.

We're not here to give you our top tips for finding your dream man or woman. That's up to you. We're more concerned that you're looking after yourself, whether you're in a relationship or not.

LOOK AFTER YOUR RELATIONSHIP

A relationship is like a living thing; it needs attention and nourishment, and it needs them regularly, not just once in a while when you remember about date night. Remember that resentment and measuring yourselves against each other will destroy a relationship – eventually, if not immediately. This applies to all relationships, not just romantic ones, although in this section we're mostly talking about a relationship with a partner.

It's easy to get complacent in a romantic relationship over time. And sometimes it can feel as if romance has left the building entirely. Try some of these ideas to nurture your relationship (you may be doing them already).

* Make sure you have proper time together, when neither of you is on your phone or watching TV. Try establishing a regular date night in the diary.

* You know how excited the dog gets when you come home? It's a great feeling to be welcomed like that, right? Can you be that happy when someone you love comes home? Show them how glad you are that they're back.

* Be respectful and kind to each other, even if you're angry (especially if you're angry).

* Give each other space to be your own person and to do the things that give you joy, whether it's hobbies or time with friends. You need time apart from each other and especially, if you have them, time apart from the kids.

* Do thoughtful things for each other. Think about what your partner needs or what makes them happy. It doesn't have to be an expensive gift; for some people it's as small as tea in bed in the morning. On days your partner is busy or getting home late, take over the cleaning and cooking. Don't just wait for special occasions to make loving gestures, whether big or small.

* If you've been together for a long time, you may assume you know how your partner is feeling. You could be wrong – ask them.

* It works the other way, too – don't assume they know what you want. People aren't telepathic. If something is bothering you, say so.

* Sex can become a source of tension in a long-term relationship. You have to figure out a way to make sure both of you are having your needs met.

* Speak to each other the way you'd like to be spoken to.

Nadia: 'In my pregnancy yoga class I do a breathing exercise where people get into pairs. One puts their hands on the other's back, to help them feel whether they're breathing deeply, right into their back ribs.'

'When it's two women who don't know each other, they speak so sweetly to one another, with big smiles, "Can you breathe a bit more deeply, just here?" But couples can snap at each other, and practically smack each other in the place they want them to breathe more! Even if you're stressed or angry, try to speak nicely to your partner, and hopefully they will do the same for you. It's a good habit.'

Katia: 'My husband Casey knows mornings are not my thing, so he goes down with the kids every morning and makes them breakfast and brings me a cup of tea in bed. It's a little thing but it reminds me all over again what a good husband I have. He knows: Happy Wife, Happy Life.'

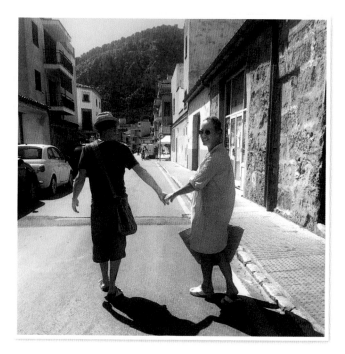

LOVING KINDNESS MEDITATION

The loving kindness meditation is a practice of directing well wishes, kindness and friendship towards yourself and others. It can get rid of built-up negative emotions in a relationship and transform how you feel about your partner and about yourself. It works with friends, colleagues and family, too.

1. Start by bringing your attention to yourself, then silently repeat these words, three times:

   May I be safe. May I be healthy. May I be happy. May I find peace.

2. Think of someone you love, where the relationship is easy and happy. Repeat to yourself:

   May you be safe. May you be healthy. May you be happy. May you find peace.

3. Think of someone neutral, perhaps a person you see daily but don't have a close relationship with – like the person at your local coffee shop or someone you see on your way to work - and repeat the words silently, directing your loving kindness to them.

4. Now repeat the same words, but send them to someone who you're having a hard time with. It can be a disagreement at work or an argument with a friend.

   It may feel difficult to do at first. If you are angry, take your time with it, and see if you can observe your feelings begin to change.

5. Then extend your loving kindness to all beings everywhere (that really means everyone – even that person on the news who makes you furious every time you see them).

   May you all be safe. May you all be healthy. May you all be happy. May you all find peace.

LETTING GO OF RESENTMENT

Most of us have plenty of things that annoy us about our partner, and we all know that sometimes it's the smallest things that cause the biggest fights.

It could be as insignificant as your partner not picking up their dirty socks when you've asked them to. Feeling as if you're being ignored can make an abandoned pair of socks feel like a personal attack.

So it may be better for you to think of the things you love about your partner, instead of the things you don't. The socks may not get picked up, but accepting that you are no longer filled with resentment about it is self-care.

This isn't about excusing disrespectful behaviour from a partner – you deserve to be treated well in a relationship – but learning to make your own peace with small annoyances is a way for you to feel better, and it may make your relationship better in turn. So, when niggles arise, stop and think:

* When you were first in love, did the socks on the floor bother you?

* Have you said clearly what you need? Have you said, 'Can I just say, it really annoys me when . . ?'

* Are you being a perfectionist and holding on to your way of doing things? Is it that big a deal in the grand scheme of things? Do you need to let it go?

* Catch yourself as you get angry about the socks. Put your anger into perspective by thinking of all the other amazing things your partner does.

* See if you can just let it go.

SUMMER ROLLS

These rice-paper rolls look as if they're super complicated, but they're actually really easy to make. They're incredibly versatile – once you've got the hang of the rolling technique you can mix up the ingredients to use whatever you have to hand. It might be leftover chicken or fish, or sliced raw vegetables.

If you can't find it at the supermarket, rice paper is worth tracking down online as it lasts in the cupboard for literally years.

Once made, these rolls dry out quite quickly, so they're best eaten within a few hours.

Makes 10

*250g cooked noodles
  (traditionally these
  are rice noodles,
  but use whatever
  you have)*

*1 tbsp tamari or light
  soy sauce*

1 tsp sesame oil

20 sheets of rice paper

*1 avocado, peeled,
  stoned and sliced*

*1 large cucumber,
  julienned*

bunch of mint leaves

*small bag of
  baby spinach*

*2 tbsp mixed black and
  white sesame seeds*

Toss the cooked noodles in the tamari or soy sauce and sesame oil and set aside.

Make the peanut sauce by blending the lime juice with the chilli and garlic – I use a blender for this but don't overblend as it's good to have a bit of texture. Stir in the remaining ingredients, adding a little more water if the sauce feels too thick.

Now, get ready to roll.

Put hot water from the tap into a frying pan and carefully place a sheet of rice paper in the water, then move it around for a few seconds until it softens. You don't want the rice paper to be too hard to fold, but you also don't want it to collapse. It may take a few attempts to find that happy medium.

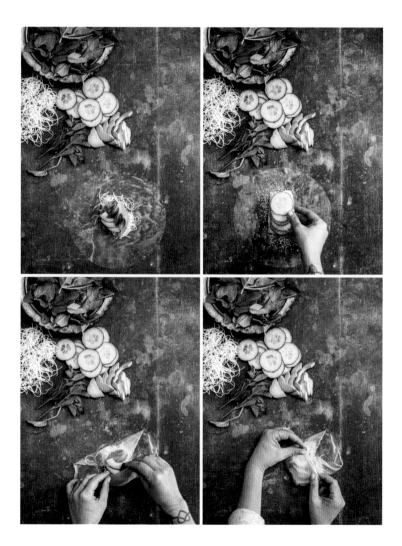

For the peanut sauce

juice of 1 lime

*½ red chilli, deseeded
and finely chopped*

*1 garlic clove, finely
chopped*

*3 tbsp crunchy
peanut butter*

2 tbsp olive oil

3 tbsp water

*2 tsp tamari or
light soy sauce*

1 tsp sesame oil

Lay your soaked rice paper on a tea towel to remove some of the water, then lay it out flat on a chopping board and get all of your ingredients assembled nearby.

Stack your first layer of filling ingredients neatly in the middle of the soft rice paper, horizontally, in this order: lay 2 slices of avocado next to each other, top with 2 cucumber strips and then add a small handful of dressed noodles, followed by 3 mint leaves and finally 5–8 baby spinach leaves.

Mould the ingredients with your hands to make a tight oval shape, then fold in the sides of the rice paper and roll up from the bottom (look at the photographs if this is confusing).

Soak another sheet of rice paper until soft, then sprinkle it with some sesame seeds. Lay your first roll in the middle of the second rice paper sheet and re-roll in the same way as before. The sesame seeds will show through the rice paper and look beautiful. Repeat to make 10 individual rolls.

If you're in a rush, just skip the second layer.

Serve with the peanut sauce on the side.

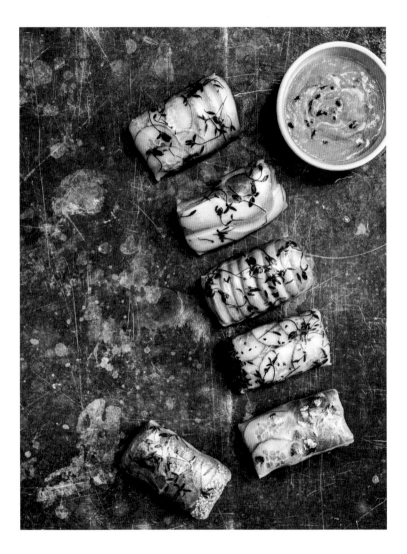

BEETROOT PÂTÉ

This is one of the recipes I created when I set up my first café thirteen years ago. It hasn't been off the menu since; people love it. It thickens overnight so it is best made the night before.

You can use this in so many ways – in a sushi roll with nori, served as a pâté with cucumber, avocado, carrot sticks and alfalfa, on toast with goat's cheese or feta and loaded with avocado and rocket for an open-faced sandwich, or simply as a dipping sauce with carrot and cucumber sticks.

Serves 4

1 red pepper, deseeded and roughly chopped

1 raw beetroot, peeled and chopped (approx. 175g)

½ red chilli, deseeded and roughly chopped

4 tbsp apple cider vinegar

1 tbsp maple syrup

2 tbsp tamari or light soy sauce

150g cashew nuts

Put everything in a blender and whiz until smooth. If you don't have a high-speed blender you may need to help the process along by stopping to stir the mixture a few times while you're blending.

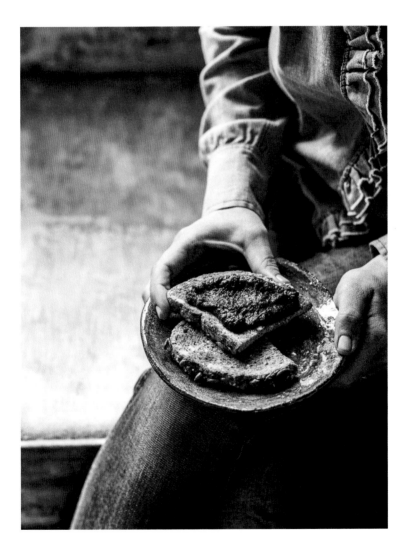

VANILLA CUSTARD TART WITH BERRIES

Makes 4 or 5 individual 10cm tarts, or 1 large 20cm tart.

For the crust
125g walnuts (soaked overnight)
125g pecans (soaked overnight)
40g chopped dried figs
1 date, stoned
pinch of salt

For the vanilla cashew cream
175g cashews (soaked for up to 4 hours)
seeds from ½ vanilla pod
6 tbsp maple syrup
6 tbsp water (adding slowly as you might not need it all)
1 drop food-grade lavender oil (optional)

For the topping
400g mixed berries
dried rose petals (optional)
dried lavender flowers (optional)

I developed this tart when I was running a café that specialised in raw food. I don't much go for super-restrictive diets these days, but I still love this recipe, and it's a great one for any dinner guest who has dietary intolerances.

Preheat the oven to 175°C/350°F/Gas mark 4 and line your tart dish or dishes with cling film. Line a baking tray with baking parchment.

Put all the crust ingredients in a food processor and pulse until you get a sticky, dough-like consistency. You may need to add a drop of water to bring it together. Press the crust mixture into the dish or dishes to make a tart case that goes up the side of the dish.

Lift the cling film to remove the moulded case from the tart dish – it should hold its shape. Remove the cling film, place the case on the baking tray and cook it for 15 minutes until golden – be careful it doesn't burn. Remove from the oven and leave to cool.

While the crust is cooling, make the vanilla cashew cream by blending all of the ingredients, plus the lavender oil if you're using it, into a smooth, custard-like consistency.

Spoon the vanilla cashew cream into the cooled tart cases and decorate with berries and dried flowers, if you like.

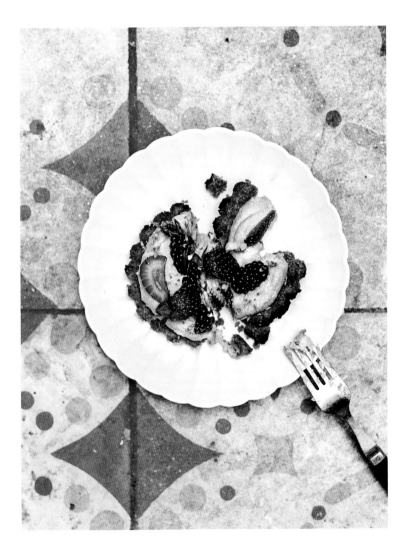

FRIENDS AND FAMILY

'If you think you are enlightened, go spend a week with your family.' *Ram Dass*

It's a truth that you can't choose your family, but you can choose your friends. If your family isn't able to give you what you need, you can create a new and more loving family amongst your friends. It's also possible to love your family but not to like them very much, or to want to spend time with them. And that is fine. We know we are very lucky to have a very close relationship, not just as sisters but also as friends, but we have had challenging relationships with other family members.

For the best self-care, all your relationships should be mutually kind and loving, with clear boundaries. It's harder to get out of a relationship with your family, but the same friendship rules apply: if you wouldn't take it from a friend, don't take it from a family member either.

Different relationships have different needs, and your relationships with everyone will change and evolve over time. Learn and notice what each relationship requires from you, and what each brings to the table for you. The energy of any relationship should feel like it flows back and forth – it's not good self-care if the flow of love and attention only goes one way. You can't expect people to be there for you if you're not going to put something back.

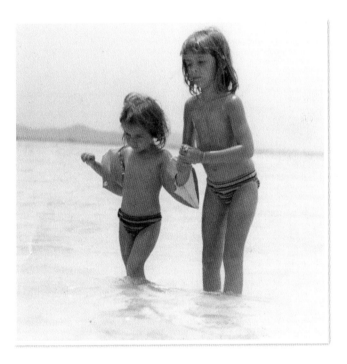

HOW TO HOLD YOUR BOUNDARIES

Have you been guilty of putting your friends or family before yourself? Of course it's important to give to others, but giving too much may make you resentful. Only give as much as you're comfortable with. Check in with yourself, paying attention to the fine line between pleasing someone else and how it makes you feel. If it doesn't feel good, you know you've hit your limit.

There will be times when you are not in the mood but you still have to make an effort for someone else. At those times, be clear about your boundaries. It's okay to say, 'I'd love to come to your party, but I can only stay an hour.' Or, 'I can help you with your house move on Tuesday, but not tomorrow.'

Remember you are a better support for a friend, family member or partner if you don't take on their problem as if it was your own. Some distance is helpful for them and also for you.

Maybe you know someone who calls you all the time to talk about the same problem? They may be asking for help, but it feels like they're not doing anything to change the situation. All you need to do is listen and be there to support and hold and love, without trying to come up with a solution or attempting to 'fix' their problem.

If you have hit a wall and can't hear it any more, be honest and tell them. You can say, 'I love you, but I don't love this situation and it is hard for me to talk to you about it right now.' They may take offence, but try to stay steady and true to what you need to look after you.

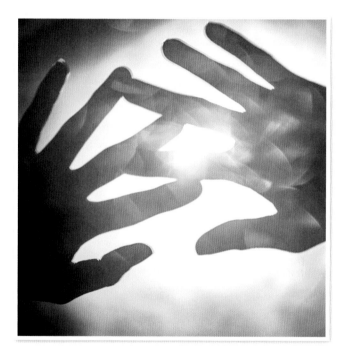

THE GOOD FRIEND GUIDE

To practise self-care, there are possibly some friends whose presence you need to limit, and some you need to see more of. Do you have any of these people in your life?

SEE MORE OF . . .

The brilliant friend. She's got your back, she's earned your trust, she's kind and she is inspirational. You can be vulnerable with her without fear of being thought needy. Hopefully your support system includes one or more people like this who you can say anything to, without having to process it first. Hang out with them at all opportunities!

The good times friend. Fun and light, she's brilliant company but she may not be there for you if you're in trouble. As long as you know that, it's fine.

The old friend. You might be lucky enough to have friends who you've known since you were a child or teenager. They might be completely different from you now in every way, but your oldest friends can often lock right into the real you. It's good to have people around you who have known you through all the different cycles of your life.

SEE SOMETIMES . . .

The heavy friend. If one of your friends is going through a lot of drama and it's too heavy for you, don't be scared to take a break from it. It's not being rude, or abandoning them, it's about protecting yourself by not engaging as much in their drama as you normally might.

The self-destructive friend. Sometimes you have a friend who is in a really bad way, maybe because of alcohol or drugs. Your boundary then is to do as much as feels right. You might go for a walk with them, or hang out with them in an environment that doesn't support the destructive behaviour. If you don't want to see them, maybe the most you can do is keep in touch via text or message, saying you're thinking of them, you're hoping they're okay, that you love them and wish them better.

SEE NEVER . . .

The friend who puts you last. If you are the last person to get the call or the invitation and the meeting is always on the other person's terms, it's perfectly acceptable to refuse it. If you are bottom of their list, it's not self-care to put that person on the top of yours. Good friends are equals in a relationship.

The friend who's not kind. There are some people you may think of as good friends but their actions don't show that. To anyone who belittles you, betrays you or hasn't got your back – goodbye!

ARE YOU REALLY FRIENDS?

If you're wondering if you should make the effort to be or stay friends with someone, ask yourself the following questions. If the answer to any of them is a 'no', this person may be an acquaintance, not a true friend. It's fine to see them if it doesn't make you feel bad, but it may not be worth investing your emotional energy in the relationship.

* Does this person make you feel uplifted and supported?

* Is silence between you comfortable?

* Would you totally trust them with a secret?

* Would that friend be there for you if you had a problem?

* Do they inspire you, or do you inspire them?

* Do they listen to what you say? Really listen?

HOW TO HELP SOMEONE IN NEED

Bad things happen to friends and family, and when they do, you will be there, but not at your own expense. Remember, you need to put on your oxygen mask first.

*   Don't feel guilt that your life is good in that moment and theirs isn't; things always change and tables always turn.

*   Share the load. If someone is in real need because of loss, divorce or illness, create a rota between all their closest people to help them out. Some people could bring food, others could sign up to sit with them at hospital appointments, and others could just visit for a chat.

*   When you can't be there, make sure your friend knows you are thinking of them. Tell them they don't have to reply to you, just keep in touch, sending cards or texts.

*   Be a good listener. Listening is an art, and it's not easy. Next time someone is talking to you, try to listen without interrupting. When someone is going through a hard time, this isn't the time to share your own experiences.

FINDING YOUR TRIBE

In the Buddhist tradition, your tribe or group of like-minded people is called your sanga. Your tribe isn't exactly the same thing as your friends, though there may be crossover; instead you'll recognise your tribe by their similar belief system or interests, maybe in healthy eating, doing yoga, learning philosophy, going to poetry readings, women's or men's groups, or whatever. Finding a tribe is self-care because it provides you with a primal feeling of belonging, which is an essential human need.

On first meeting, your tribe may not appear to be anything like you. But you may find you have a deeper connection that's less about where you come from or what you look like and more about beliefs, a similar moral code or mind-set or shared human experiences.

What unites people can be stronger than their differences. When you do things that are about the essence of you – whether it's going to a pottery class or an AA meeting – you'll find the people who get you. You'll feel you can be open, honest and vulnerable with your tribe.

There are also tribes that form because of situation. Those may be your work friends or your parent friends. You may not have as much in common in terms of interest or even outlook, but the constant sharing – the giving and taking that you each do – gives you a bond and creates trust. When someone is a member of your tribe, you don't feel scared to ask for help because you know you would do the same for them.

HOW TO NURTURE YOUR TRIBE

* Make the effort to get together regularly. It can become harder to keep your community together as life brings more responsibilities. Plan once a month or at least every few months to meet or you'll get so busy you'll never see each other.

  If you don't spend time together, you won't know what's happening in each other's lives and you'll lose those touchstones that are so vital. Even if you become a parent or get promoted or move away, it's good to be reminded of the person you were.

* Really listen. Are you too quick to jump in with your stories? Consciously try not to talk over anyone and not to interrupt. Hold the space so you're listening, then you will be heard too.

* Have shared experiences that will make memories. Have dinner together rather than going to the pub, so you can talk properly.

* Hang out in a group of only women (if you're a woman) or only men (if you're a man). We're not talking about parties, stag or hen dos; gatherings of solely men and women have been going on for centuries. They provide an opportunity for women and men to be completely themselves and to be able to address issues that solely affect them.

* Receive as well as give. Be happy to ask for and accept help. It feels nice to be given the opportunity to help someone and it strengthens your group bonds.

HOW TO BOND WITH A NEW TRIBE

What are your interests? What fires you up? What do you love doing? What makes you feel good? It might be that you have found a passion for, say, cooking or yoga or hiking, but your family and friends aren't on the same trip. You can't force people to get into what you like.

Sometimes you need to get out there and find the people who love the things that you do. And not just online – here's how to bond in real life.

* Find people who like what you do. It could be a cookery class, or being on the local council, or volunteering for a charity. Once you know what does it for you and you find a group who share the same interests, you will most likely be surrounded by likeminded people: your tribe.

* Over time you will get to know them. So, for example, if you are into yoga, you will start talking to people from the class you attend. Then you might go to a talk together, or a workshop, or go on retreat. It's doing activities together that forms the strongest bonds.

* Share with the group. Acknowledging a shared experience, whether through talking or through a simple ritual, can be powerful.

> Nadia: 'There's a bonding exercise I do towards the end of a yoga retreat or a workshop. We get into a circle, and as we go around the group each person shares something they feel grateful for learning or experiencing on the retreat. Then we each take a piece of red string, turn to the person next to us and tie it around their wrist. After the retreat, that red string is a reminder of the week together and the experience we shared.'

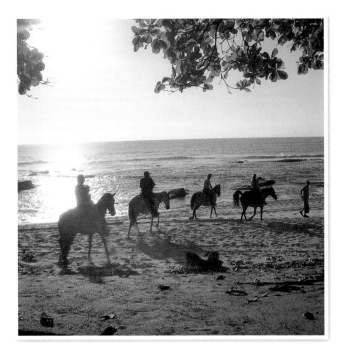

LETTING GO

'Like a leaf falling from a tree, she just let go. There was no effort.
There was no struggle. It wasn't good and it wasn't bad. It was what
it was, and it is just that.' *Ernest Holmes*

There's one change you can make that will shift your whole life: let go.

Are you a self-confessed control freak? Do you strive to nail the job, the outfit or the parenting every time? It's really, really hard to do it all. And if you never let up, something's going to give: you are exhausting yourself.

If you are reading this and you're not a control freak, you probably don't get why people get stressed about little things. But if you are one, it can feel like every cell in your body is in code red when your partner gets the wrong dessertspoons out!

Don't worry: letting go is not about no longer caring, it's realising that sometimes things can be good enough because you're good enough. We're not saying don't work bloody hard, just don't beat yourself up if the result isn't perfect.

The key to letting go is finding an inner feeling of self-contentment, no matter what. People will still love you if you're not perfect. Think of your friends: it's probably their imperfections and quirks that you love most about them.

Is your need to get things right based on fear of failure? The funny thing is, perfectionists often make mistakes because they're driving themselves too hard. Perfectionism is the opposite of joy. When you accept life isn't perfect, you can relax into it.

Nadia: 'I used to be a perfectionist, and it stopped me from doing things because I was afraid. I was afraid to speak out because I was afraid I'd fail. I needed to prove myself with anything I did. As I got older, I came to see that some of the things I do well now are because I messed them up first.'

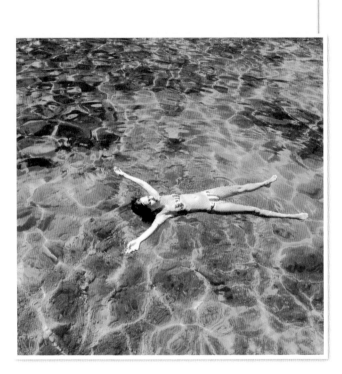

HOW TO FORGIVE (YOURSELF)

Okay, so you've behaved badly. You were unkind to your mum on the phone. Or perhaps you did something embarrassing, such as texting an ex? Or awful, such as revealing a friend's secret? Before you punish yourself, work through the situation calmly.

* Notice when you're feeling bad and when you think it might be (somewhat) your fault.

* Ask yourself: do I need to apologise to someone? If the answer is yes, just go and do it. Most people will appreciate a real apology. Don't worry about whether that person is going to forgive you or like you afterwards – you can't control that.

* Be clear what your part was in the incident, and think about why you behaved like that. Don't try to justify your behaviour, just question it.

* Don't lay all the blame on the other person.

* Show yourself some compassion – were you acting out of fear, or anger or sadness? We all make mistakes, so be kind, rather than judgemental.

* Let it go. Even if you're not forgiven, you need to let it go.

LEARNING TO BE FLEXIBLE

You might find that there's a particular area where your anxiety and fear drive you and you just cannot let go. Maybe it's that your home needs to be utterly clean at every moment, or that you over deliver at work because you can't bear not to be the best at everything.

You can pretty much guarantee that things in life aren't going to go exactly as you want them to. That is not a problem in itself, that is just the experience of being human in the world. How you deal with this is the problem, and the solution is to lessen your grip and start to let go.

How can you let go? The first step is paying attention when you feel yourself holding too tight to a situation or an outcome.

* Notice your intention. If you're cooking a meal for others, is it to give everyone a beautiful experience or to have praise for yourself at the end of it? If you're clinging too tightly to a romantic relationship, is it because you love this person, or because you want people to think of you as part of the perfect couple?

* Notice when you start to feel agitated or begin to get worked up that things aren't exactly how you want or would do them.

* Once you start to notice the feeling, tell yourself 'it's no big deal'. This will be tough at first, but keep reminding yourself, until you begin to believe it.

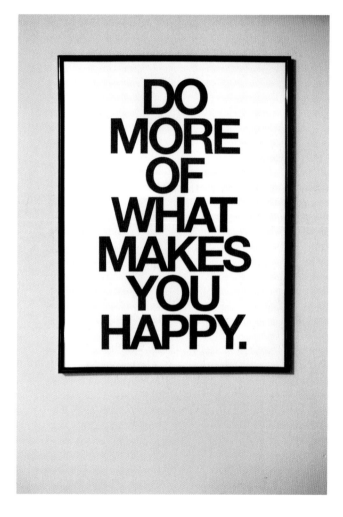

BE AN INSPIRATION,
NOT A PREACHER

Okay, so you've found your healthy life: a way of eating that makes you feel full of energy and an exercise regime that makes you feel strong. We're super happy for you, but please don't start preaching to all your friends and family. Constantly talking about how healthy and amazing we are can make others feel judged and bad about themselves. Wellbeing is not a competition; we're all on our own path.

In particular, don't force your partner to change with you. When you fell in love maybe you both used to go out for dinner and dancing, or get a bit tipsy together. Now you want to do your new thing: yoga, eating paleo or vegan, taking part in triathlons or ditching alcohol, and you want them to do it too. Is that fair? It's as unfair for you to take all the sugar out of the house, for example, as it would be for your partner to smoke in the house, if that's what you hate.

If you are eating celery sticks and drinking a cup of hot water with lemon at dinner, don't force everyone to do that (also, why are you doing that?). Live by example: cook great food, show people you're happier and healthier, don't tell them so.

When you feel good and look good, people will want a part of that.

WHEN YOUR JOY
FEELS FAR AWAY

'You cannot protect yourself from sadness without protecting yourself from happiness.' *Jonathan Safran Foer*

It's normal to feel low every now and again – whether it's because of your hormones, or an illness or the comedown after a big event. Then there are the triggers you have even less control over: something you care about goes wrong, you feel you've failed at work, the news cycle is overwhelming.

When you feel low, it's crucial to practise self-care, even if it's the last thing you feel like doing. Do something, however small: meditate, get out into nature, eat something nourishing. Try anything that will keep you engaged and uplifted, so you don't sink into your feelings.

We're not saying self-care should replace seeing a health professional, like a doctor or therapist. In fact, we are big fans of therapy and would recommend it to anyone and everyone who is going through any difficulty.

But, as you probably know, some of the things we love to recommend in self-care – exercise, for one – are part of a whole host of lifestyle changes recommended by doctors to lift mood. Self-care is not a cure, but it may help you press pause on a downward cycle and give you a bit of space to breathe outside it.

Feeling low means different things to different people: maybe you sleep too much or don't sleep at all. Perhaps you don't look forward to things or feel there's no meaning to what you do. Or you get short tempered, or worry more.

The one thing that is almost always true for a low mood is that you can't see outside it when you're in it. You might feel defeated. You might not want to get out of bed, or if you do, you may have no enthusiasm for the day ahead.

It might be that the best self-care at these times in your life is about recognising it's important for you to be sad right now. Maybe you need to allow yourself time to heal and be in those feelings before you can move on from them. What would you tell someone you really care about, if he or she felt like this?

Or perhaps feeling low has become a habit and you're always waiting for someone or something else to rescue you or change you so you're finally happy. What small changes can you make to rescue yourself, instead of waiting for someone else to do it?

> Nadia: 'I used to be always waiting for something to change so that I could be happy. I only knew high drama and longing for what I didn't have. The three things that made a difference were: a daily gratitude practice (see page 74), meditating daily and being consistent about seeing a therapist every week. For the past few years, I have consistently felt joyful and contented, the longest stretch ever in my life, for no apparent reason. When I used to feel low I'd think, am I ever going to get out of this? But now I know the feelings won't last, they will pass.'

WHY WE LOVE THERAPY

Therapy is life-changing and powerful, and it almost always puts you on a better footing with life.

What you get in that room, from that relationship with a person who starts out as a stranger, is very different from the support you get from a friend or family member (although that is invaluable, too). In therapy, you get to talk, all of the time, about you, without fear of offending someone or boring them or embarrassing yourself.

A good therapist can help you see your life from the outside and can pick up on things you didn't know you were thinking or doing. Therapy gives you unwavering support and a new way of understanding how you relate to the world and yourself.

It's important to understand that having therapy does not mean there is something wrong with you; it is just a way to help you see familiar situations from a new perspective.

Yes, it's expensive, but when we feel the need for therapy we'd rather have it over new shoes or a night out. Just a few sessions can make a big difference, especially if you are going through something major in your life.

You do need to find the right therapist, though. It's best to have a personal recommendation, but if you don't have that, see a few and find one who sits right with you.

Back in the day, people facing a problem might have gone to see their priest, or their rabbi, or perhaps a village chief; a therapist is just the modern, secular solution to some of the age-old issues of being human.

Don't be afraid to ask for help.

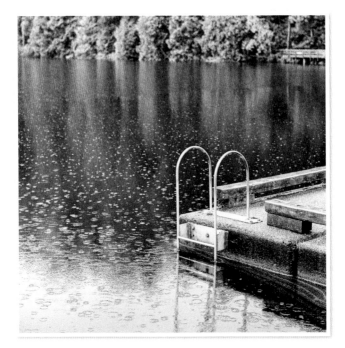

GET OUT OF YOUR HEAD AND INTO YOUR BODY

Find a way to step outside the repetitive cycle of your thoughts and you will start to see yourself from the outside, with a bit more perspective. This is true whether you're feeling bad, sad or anxious. You may have to force yourself to do it; we promise it's worth it.

* Do any task that requires concentration and focus. This will shift you out of the repeating circuits of your mind. Try learning something new, whether it's painting, learning an instrument or a new language.

* Do something that involves moving your body as well as concentration, such as skateboarding, cycling, walking or a yoga class (or try the yoga for calm exercise on the next page).

* Watch some comedy. Even in the most cynical mood, you might be able to find a comedy that's dark enough to make you laugh. Proper laughing out loud floods your body with happy hormones; even a wry smile is better than nothing.

* Change the scenery. Go for a walk somewhere new, it doesn't have to be far away, maybe just a different neighbourhood. New sights and experiences will change your thought cycle, even if only temporarily.

* Staying in with only your thoughts for company can send you on a downward spiral. Break the spiral by getting out and seeing the people who support you, whether you need a laugh or a cry.

YOGA FOR CALM

Sit on the ground (or a cushion, yoga block or bolster if you prefer) with your legs crossed and your spine straight.

Slowly roll your head three times in a circle. Keep your shoulders relaxed and your jaw soft. Notice any tension in the neck or shoulders.

Roll your head three times in the opposite direction.

Fold forwards, over your crossed legs, to stretch the spine. Extend the arms in front of you.

Come back up, change the cross of your legs (so the right shin goes in front of the left shin, or vice versa), and fold forwards again.

Come onto your hands and knees with your back in a tabletop position.

Arch, then curl your spine gently and slowly a few times. Notice how your body feels.

Sit backwards so your bottom is on your heels, then fold your body forwards into child's pose. You can rest your forehead on the ground or on a block or cushion. You can have your arms straight out or down by your sides, whichever is most comfortable for you. Rest for a few breaths.

Sit up onto your bottom, with your legs stretched out in front of you.

Bend your left knee out to the side, placing the left foot on the inside of the right thigh.

Keeping your right leg straight, reach your arms up, then reach forwards for your right foot or ankle, or rest your arms alongside your right leg.

Take three to five breaths.

As you inhale, come up to sitting.

Now extend your left leg and bend the right, and repeat on the other side.

As you inhale, come up to sitting.

Lie on your back with your feet flat on the ground, a little wider than hips. Let your knees drop together so they touch.

Put your right hand on your belly and your left hand on your chest.

Take slow, steady breaths, counting in for four and out for four, feeling the breath rise from your belly to your chest.

Then count your breath in for four, out for six.

Finally, count in for four, out for eight.

Let your breathing return to its normal rhythm, then lie down fully and let your whole body relax into the ground for two minutes.

HOW TO STOP YOUR THOUGHTS SNOWBALLING

You know how it goes, you start with a small worry and before you know it you're overcome with giant, uncomfortable thoughts. Maybe you have to have a difficult conversation with someone and you wind yourself up for days with all the possible outcomes (most of them terrible). What if the conversation turns out to be way easier than you imagined? You'll have wasted all your time and energy on nothing.

Small anxieties can lead us downwards into another layer of even bigger ones, such as 'I feel bad and I'm going to feel this awful for the rest of my life'. No, you aren't: you are going to learn to manage your mind.

We like to describe what's happening to your thoughts as a snowball rolling down a hill, growing and growing as it collects more snow.

The first step to stopping this is simply to notice when an uncomfortable thought arises. Take a breath and see if you can create a bit of space between your thoughts.

Ask yourself: is this thought a fact, or is it my interpretation? Where does it come from? Is it an old story I often tell myself, for example, that people always leave me?

As you watch and observe your thoughts, bring yourself back to being present in the situation as it stands, as opposed to what your thoughts have created.

You've stopped the snowball.

CALMING ALTERNATE-NOSTRIL BREATHING

This is a yogic breathing technique that helps to calm the mind and release stress. It's said to balance the right and left sides of the brain. It's certainly very good for helping you feel balanced physically, mentally and emotionally.

Try it the next time you feel your thoughts running away with you.

1. Sit either on a chair with your feet on the ground, or cross-legged on the floor, propped up on a cushion. If you are on a chair, take your shoes off so you can feel the ground.

2. Begin to connect to your breathing. Start with slow, smooth steady breaths. You may already start to feel your body relax.

3. Rest your left hand on your left knee with the palm facing up, the tip of the index finger and tip of the thumb touching.

4. Take your right hand and bend the index and middle fingers towards the palm. You are going to use the thumb to block the right nostril and the ring finger to block the left nostril.

5. First, block the right nostril with the thumb lightly and breathe in and out through your left nostril a few times.

6. Next, release the right nostril and block the left nostril with the ring finger. Breathe in and out through the right nostril.

7. Block the right nostril and inhale through the left nostril to a count of four. Then block the left nostril and exhale from the right nostril to a count of eight.

   Inhale through the right nostril to a count of four, then block the right nostril and exhale from the left to a count of eight. This is one round.

9. Continue for five full rounds. Once you've done this, release your hands.

10. Breathing through both nostrils, sit quietly for a couple of minutes and notice how you feel.

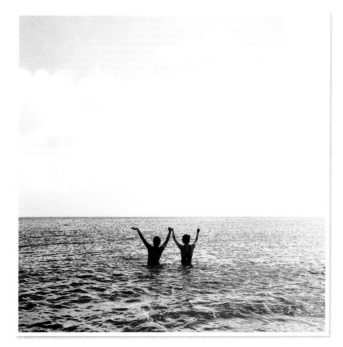

HOW TO BRING
MORE JOY
INTO YOUR LIFE

* Check in with yourself. Notice how you feel. Do this every day, a few times a day if you can.

* Ask yourself, what does joy feel like to you? When did you last experience joy?

* When do you feel you are not aligned with the feeling of joy? How can you address this, to feel better?

* Ask yourself, what would joy feel like right now in this moment?

* What could you do, right now, to feel more joyful?

* Do something for yourself today that brings you a sense of joyfulness.

light

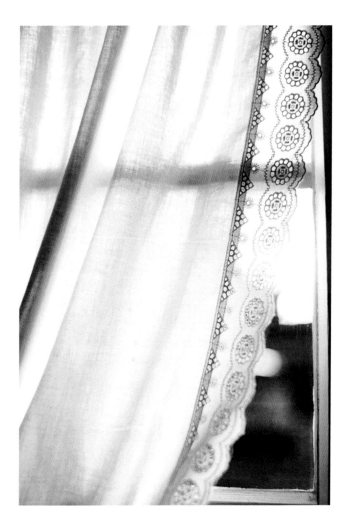

'As we let our own light shine, we unconsciously give other people permission to do the same. As we are liberated from our own fear, our presence automatically liberates others.'
Marianne Williamson

Have you ever seen a friend who seems to be lit from within? Or said of someone that their eyes 'lit up'? Even people who shy away from any talk of spirituality use light as a metaphor for the energy force that is in us all. When you feel vibrant and energised, it is visible to everyone. Another way of describing your light is your life force; in Chinese medicine it's called your chi, and in yoga it's called your prana. Your light sustains you from the inside.

Your light dims when you feel low or unwell, when you're stressed or traumatised. It gets even lower if you don't look after yourself. People pay so much attention to their skincare or their clothes, but it's your inner light that is most attractive to others. When your light is bright, people see you shine, no matter what you're wearing.

This section is about how to ignite and nurture the light within, whether that's first thing in the morning or last thing at night, at home or away. Make checking in to your energy a regular part of your day – don't decide to wait for a less busy time, or a holiday, or a weekend. If you take care of your energy whenever you have the opportunity, you can feel good wherever you go.

May your force be with you.

START THE DAY RIGHT

'Every morning, when we wake up, we have 24 brand new hours to live. What a precious gift! We have the capacity to live in a way that these 24 hours will bring peace, joy, and happiness to ourselves and others.' *Thich Nhat Hanh*

How does your day usually start? Are you woken suddenly by being jumped on by a child, cat or dog? Do you roll over, pick up your phone and read the news, or check Twitter or Instagram? Do you hit the snooze button over and over? If so, you are setting up your body and mind to be reactive, rather than getting yourself in a good space before your day begins.

We want to help you find a way to wake up gently, and to choose for yourself how you approach the day. Starting the morning in the right way allows you to feel calm and spacious, rather than jolted and jittery. Taking an early moment for yourself will help you have perspective all day, so you can respond to whatever events arise rather than react to them.

Before you get out of bed:

* Write a super-quick gratitude list. It could be as simple as being grateful for the bed you've slept in or as big as the roof over your head. You could even write down what you find challenging then say 'thank you for that lesson I learnt', or 'thank you, I now know how to deal with that difficult situation differently'.

* Read a page from an inspirational book first thing, rather than getting immersed in the news as soon as you wake up.

*   Set an intention for the day. Think, or write down, how you want your day to feel. For example, 'I am energised and inspired for the day ahead'.

*   Send a loving text to someone. It could be a thank you, an offer of help or just an 'I love you'.

*   Have a hug. It might sound corny, but whether it comes from your dog, cat, partner or child, a hug is pure joy. It increases your levels of oxytocin, the love hormone.

*   Check in to see how you are. You can't begin to practise self-care until you begin to notice that you're tired, or you're running on empty and have barely slept. Or perhaps you're in a bad mood – everyone has shitty days. If you don't check in, you may beat yourself up for not being on top form, or blame the world or other people for your mood. But if you notice how you are, you can deal with it – maybe by planning a walk in fresh air to wake you at lunchtime, or by packing some healthy snacks to keep you off the sugar. You can scale down your expectations of what you need to get done. And be kind to yourself.

UPGRADE YOUR MORNINGS

This is a long list, and we're not suggesting that you try all of these at once! However, start making one of these suggestions a regular habit and you may find it will transform your whole day.

* Before your morning tea or coffee, drink a cup of hot water with a slice of lemon in it, to rehydrate you, start your digestion and get your liver working.

* Set your alarm 30 minutes earlier than the rest of your household gets up. You could use the time to have a longer shower than normal, or to take some exercise. You may discover this is your most productive time for making plans or being creative. By the time the rest of the house wakes up, you'll be thinking, let's do this!

* Meditate for five to ten minutes. Just prop yourself up on your pillows so you're upright (make sure you're not so comfortable that you fall back asleep).

* Try oil pulling with coconut oil; a traditional Ayurvedic treatment for oral health that's even reputed to whiten teeth. It's easy to do: when you wake up and go to the bathroom, just put a teaspoon of coconut oil in your mouth and let it melt. Don't put in too much at once or you may feel like gagging. Switch on the kettle and, in the time it takes to boil, swill the oil around your mouth, swishing it between your teeth. Then spit the oil into the bin (never down the sink as it will block the pipes).

* Add greens to your breakfast, whether it's a side of spinach, avo on your toast, kale or spinach in your smoothie, asparagus to dip into your boiled egg or a sprinkle of parsley or coriander on your scrambled eggs.

* Do a twist to wake up your spine. Lie on your back and bring your right knee into your chest. Then cross your right knee over to the left side of your body, towards the floor. Hold the knee down with your left hand and extend your right arm out to the side, in line with your shoulder. Take three to five breaths. Repeat on the other side.

* Move for ten minutes. Whether it's doing a few moves you remember from your yoga class, having a dance around the house or a walk around the block. You've got ten minutes, surely?

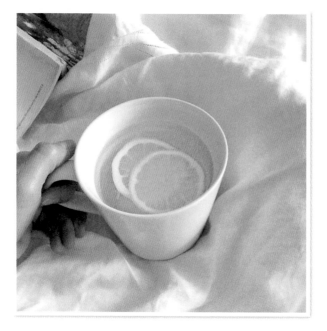

NADIA'S FIVE-MINUTE MORNING YOGA

Use this practice to check in with where your body is today.

Start standing with your feet hip distance apart. Swing your arms from side to side, breathing in and breathing out.

Bending your knees, begin to do a light bounce through your body to get the circulation going.

Then stretch your arms over your head. Hold your left wrist with your right hand, then bend to the right and feel the stretch on your left side.

Inhale and move back to the centre.

Change sides, so you hold your right wrist with your left hand, and bend over to the left.

Inhale back to the centre and release the hands.

Place your hands on your lower back and lift up your chest to the sky, arching the back.

Come onto your hands and knees. Inhale and lift the chest and seat, looking up to the sky and letting your back go concave. Then exhale to arch and round the back, looking down towards your belly. Repeat three times.

Straighten your legs to raise your bum and come into a downward dog position, keeping your knees slightly bent. Bend each knee in turn to tread from one foot to another. Then bend both knees more and raise your bum to stretch out the lower back.

Kepping your knees soft, walk your hands towards your feet. Hold each elbow and hang over your legs, keeping your knees bent. Rock a little from side to side and feel the back release.

Release your arms and roll up slowly.

Reach your arms up and over your head and hold for four counts.

Exhale for four counts as you bring your arms down.

Repeat three times.

Feel great all day.

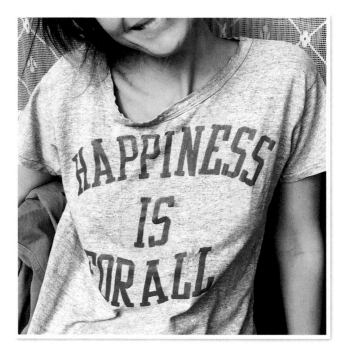

SELF-CARE IN THE WORKPLACE

'Follow the 3 Rs: Respect for self. Respect for others. Responsibility for all your actions.' *H. Jackson Brown, Jr*

At work, you're not only under stress from deadlines and targets but also from people. You're spending the day in a space shared by a lot of different people with a lot of different agendas. As well as experiencing your own emotions, you have to negotiate everyone else's too.

The most important thing you can do for workplace self-care is to check in with yourself every morning. If you're aware that you've woken up in a bad mood, perhaps you can find a way to address it before you get to the office. If you're feeling sad or really stressed, could you ask your colleagues to give you some space today? Knowing where you're at before you encounter others allows you to act out of consideration for them, as well as for yourself.

You may be lucky enough to have fantastic colleagues, but even in the best workplace environment it's likely there will be someone or something that pushes your buttons. We hope our ideas will help you not only protect your energy, but deal with all the different people and stresses.

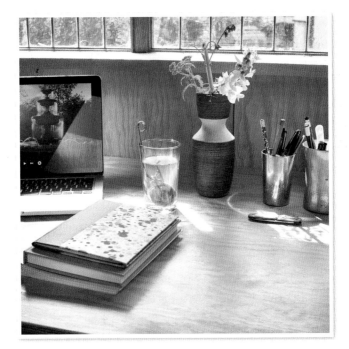

HOW TO KEEP YOUR SANITY AT WORK

* To counteract all the sitting you do at work, try to get moving before you arrive at the office. Get off the bus a few stops early, or walk up the escalator instead of standing on it.

* If it's appropriate in your workplace, wear headphones and listen to some calming music at your desk. If you find it hard to concentrate, see if music without words is better. Headphones are a sign for people to stay away, so use them with caution – don't wear them all the time, or you'll miss out on what is happening around you.

* Invest in some Chinese stress balls – two stone orbs that you circle around in your hands to calm you.

* Have a plant on your desk to look after, or fresh flowers. Any green is soothing.

* Check in with your mood regularly. Have you eaten properly? Have you drunk enough water?

* Download a web browser that tells you when to take a regular break, or gives you a positive affirmation.

* Put a crystal on your desk: quartz is beautiful to look at and is thought to be great for focus.

* Go for a walk at lunchtime and leave your work phone on your desk; plan your route and make it somewhere different each day, if you can.

* Get some fresh air. It's hard in some offices, but keep a window open if possible.

* Avoid heavy, carb-filled lunches that will make you feel sleepy.

* Keep hydrated. Put a jug of water on your desk. Add a slice of lemon, or a drop of fresh lemon oil to it to make it very refreshing (it has to be food-grade oil).

* Keep your desk really clean and tidy.

* Get as much natural light as you can, or buy a salt lamp for your desk; it's a natural air ionizer.

* Take your shoes off at work so both feet are on the floor and you can move your toes. It's good to feel your feet planted on the ground; it helps with posture, too.

* Check in with your posture every hour or so: sit up, feet on the floor, and take a few deep breaths; open up from collarbone to collarbone, and make sure your chin isn't collapsing forwards and your jaw is relaxed. This relaxes your shoulders and gives your lungs, digestive system and organs room to work.

* Try to get up from your desk every hour, even if it's just to have a walk around the office and stretch your legs.

* Put a drop of lemon oil in your palms, or on a tissue and inhale deeply. This is great for the 4pm energy slump – the scent helps with focus and keeping the mind clear.

AVOIDING THE OFFICE
SUGAR TRAP

When you're bored, does your attention stray towards the office stash of biscuits or the doughnuts a colleague brought in? So often we eat these 'treats' because we're fed up or tired rather than hungry. Instead of eating, maybe you need a break? Take a walk or make a call to a friend.

If everyone in your office agrees, can you have a week or even a month of no sugar in the office? Maybe you could bring in healthier options like the raw coco bites on page 234.

* Start a work healthy lunch club, so you all bring in something homemade and lay it out like a buffet in the office kitchen. It doesn't have to be every day, it could be every Friday. Do this and you'll all start motivating each other; you might start exercising together, or juicing, or whatever works for you.

* Have a bowl of fresh fruit on your desk. People may tease you about it, but they will help themselves, and so will you.

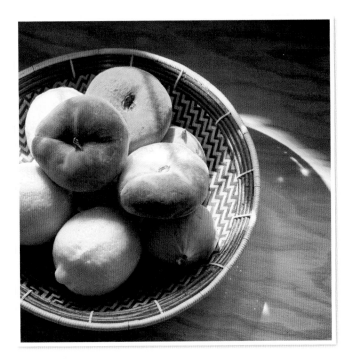

OFFICE YOGA

It helps if you have a private office for this, but even if you don't, it's worth a few funny looks to get your stretch on.

Before you start, sit on the edge of your chair, place your feet on the ground and straighten your spine as tall as possible.

Take some deep breaths.

Check in with your posture, to make sure you're not holding any tension anywhere in the body.

A spinal twist

Place your arms by your sides. As you inhale, raise your arms up and above your head.

As you exhale, twist to the right, lowering your arms so that your left hand touches your right knee and your right hand touches the chair behind your back. Look over the right shoulder.

As you inhale, raise your arms up and come back to the centre.

As you exhale, twist to your left; lower your right hand onto your left knee and rest your left hand on the chair behind your back. Look over your left shoulder.

Repeat the whole move twice.

A shoulder stretch

Sitting in your chair, raise your arms up as you inhale.

Interlace your fingers above you, with your palms facing the ceiling. Reach your palms forward as you round your back and let your head drop.

As you inhale, raise your palms up to the ceiling again.

Repeat the whole move three times.

A hip stretch

Sitting on a chair with your left foot flat on the ground (knee bent at a right angle), cross your right ankle over your left knee.

Flex the right foot and press your right knee towards the ground, so you're making a triangle shape with your legs.

Place your right elbow on your right knee and your left elbow on your right ankle.

Bring palms together in a prayer position and lean forward over your legs, lengthening the chest forward. You should feel the stretch in your right hip.

Take five breaths.

Change sides and do the whole move on the other side.

Another shoulder stretch

Sitting on the edge of your chair, separate your legs, hip width apart, with your feet firmly on the floor.

Interlace your hands behind your back and exhale as you fold forward, dropping your head between your knees and lifting your clasped hands up to the ceiling.

Hold for five breaths.

Release your arms and roll up slowly.

Scrunch all the muscles in your body and face, making fists with your hands, tightening your buttocks.

As you exhale, let everything go with a loud sigh (stick out your tongue and let out a loud roar or sigh for extra effect, though we admit this may be too much for an open-plan office!).

Repeat the whole move three times.

Desk nap

If you need a little rest, put your phone on aeroplane mode and set an alarm (a gentle chime) for 5 to 10 minutes later.

Place a pillow (or a folded coat or jacket) on your desk.

Push your chair back a little.

Lean forward, stacking your hands on the pillow and resting your forehead on your hands.

Make sure your shoulders are relaxed and your spine is in a comfortable position, with your feet on the ground.

Hope your boss isn't walking past right now . . .

PROTECTIVE ENERGY SHIELDS FOR DIFFICULT SITUATIONS

When there is something or someone in your daily life that leaves you feeling drained and negative and you really can't avoid the person or the situation, try creating an energy shield around yourself. It sounds a little out there, but think about it – if you can feel your energy being drained by a situation, why shouldn't you also be able to feel your energy being protected from it?

* Imagine a bubble of golden light surrounding and protecting you. Then take a few deep breaths inside your bubble.

* Visualise a protective sleeping bag and imagine yourself getting into it then zipping yourself up from the ground to the top of your head.

* Wash your hands after being with a difficult person, and always shower or bathe at the end of a tricky day. Water has such a powerful effect, especially if someone or something is weighing heavily on you.

* Physically grab at the space around you, imagining you're grabbing energy, and throw it away (maybe wait until your difficult person has left, so they don't see you do this!). As you do it, think of taking bad energy and flicking it off your fingertips onto the ground.

* Put a drop of lemon or peppermint essential oils onto one palm and rub your hands together. Put your nose into your cupped hands and take three deep breaths. This is good after you've been in a crowd or on public transport.

RAW COCO BITES

These are a bestseller at the café – we can't roll them fast enough! Perfect for an office snack if you're trying to resist the usual biscuits and chocolate.

Makes about 30 bites

6 Medjool dates, stoned

8 dried figs

75g desiccated coconut

110g ground almonds

3 tbsp almond butter

2 tbsp raw cacao powder

1 tbsp coconut oil

¼ tsp vanilla essence

1½ tsp maple syrup

¼ tsp salt

For dusting

1 tbsp raw cacao powder

1 tbsp desiccated coconut

1 tbsp sesame seeds

Soak the dates and figs in a bowl of just-boiled water for 5 minutes. When you drain the fruit, keep the soaking water as you may need it later.

Whiz the coconut and ground almonds in a food processor until they're really fine and powdery, then add all the remaining ingredients. Process until all the ingredients start to come together.

Slowly add some of the fig and date soaking water, 1 tablespoon at a time, and keep blending until you get a really sticky dough that forms a ball in the processor.

Roll the sticky mixture into walnut-sized balls.

Place the cacao powder, desiccated coconut and sesame seeds in three separate bowls and roll the balls in the dustings to coat completely – you can roll in just one or a mixture of all three looks lovely.

Place the balls on a plate, cover with cling film and place in the fridge overnight – they're best when they've had time to set. They can be kept for up to a week in the fridge, but there's no way they'll last that long once people have tried them!

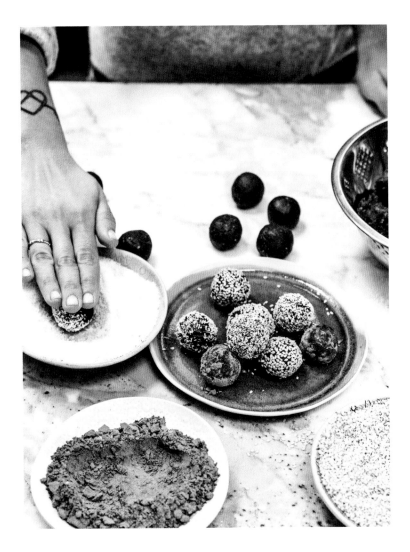

KALE, RED ONION AND SQUASH FRITTATA MUFFINS

At the café we sometimes make these with cherry tomatoes, feta and spinach instead. The beauty of this recipe is that it's so adaptable.

Makes 8 muffins

1 tbsp olive oil

2 small red onions, cut in half and sliced

250g squash, peeled and grated (I find it quickest to do this in the food processor)

150g kale leaves, finely chopped

black pepper

pinch of chilli flakes (optional)

½ tsp salt

6 eggs

1 tsp baking powder

You will need: 12-hole muffin tin and 8 paper cases.

Preheat the oven to 190°C/360°F/Gas mark 5, and put 8 paper cases into your muffin tin.

Set a deep pan on a low heat and add the olive oil. Tip in the sliced onions and let them sweat, stirring occasionally, for 10–15 minutes, until they are translucent and not browned.

Add the grated squash to the onions and cook for 5 minutes, then add the kale with a dash of black pepper, the chilli flakes, if using, and half of the salt. Cook for another 3–5 minutes, until the vegetables are soft, then switch off the heat and allow the mix to cool slightly.

Whisk the eggs in a bowl with the baking powder, a sprinkle of pepper and the rest of the salt until the mixture is pale and fluffy.

Add the cooled squash and kale mixture to the eggs and gently combine. The mixture doesn't have to be totally cold here, just move quickly if it's warm otherwise the eggs will start to scramble.

Fill each paper case almost to the top (leave some room for the muffins to rise) and cook for 20 minutes in the oven. The muffins should be nicely risen, firmed up and golden on the top.

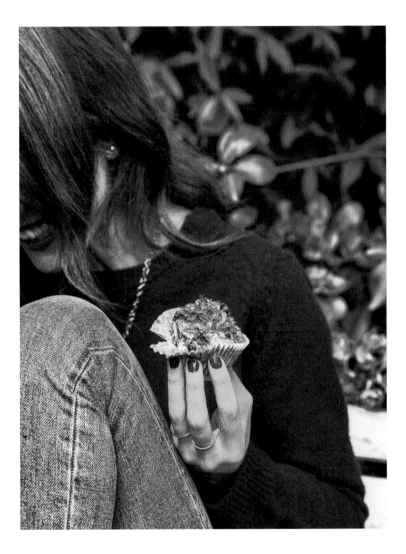

THE STAY-WELL
TRAVEL GUIDE

'Wanna fly? You've got to give up that shit that
weighs you down.' *Toni Morrison*

We're assuming you know how to manage your commute to work, if you have one, but sometimes we have to travel further afield, and it can be pretty exhausting, whether you're travelling for business or just for fun.

We've spent a lot of our lives travelling, and these are some of the tips that we've found work best for us.

ON THE PLANE

* Set your watch to the time zone of your destination as soon as you board the plane. Try to eat and sleep according to this time zone.

* Give the pre-packaged plane food a miss and bring a meal (or two) to eat instead. It can be as simple as granola with yogurt, or brown rice with cooked vegetables. It's hard to digest food during a flight, so choose something cooked (not raw) with minimal salt added. If you can't pack anything in advance, eat well before you leave home or at an airport restaurant.

* Bring your own soft blanket or a big scarf to put over your head, as well as a neck pillow, an eye mask, ear plugs or noise-cancelling headphones.

* Shake a few drops of aromatherapy oils into a little water to use as a spray. Be considerate of your neighbours and use the spray under your blanket! We use frankincense, lemon, tea tree or lavender (or a mixture) and spray this on the seats, the hand rest, the blankets – or spray on a tissue and use the tissue to wipe down the surfaces.

* It's not great to watch a film as soon as you get on the plane. See if you can relax and take a rest first, because you've probably experienced a certain amount of stress preparing for your trip and getting to the airport. It's better to rest or to fall asleep naturally then watch something afterwards, when you wake up.

* Drink water, water, water.

* It's always good to stretch out your body on the plane. Stand up by the toilets for a while and stretch out every part of you:

Rise up on your toes 15 times.

Rotate your ankles five times each way.

Stretch your quads by bending your knee behind you and reaching back for your foot.

Swing each leg a few times to each side.

Rotate your neck three times each way.

Roll your shoulders three times forwards and backwards.

Roll your head down and let your spine follow, keeping your knees bent until your hands touch the ground. Then roll back up, vertebra by vertebra. Do that three times.

WHAT TO EAT WHEN YOU'RE
ON THE MOVE

Be realistic. Travelling is stressful and this is not the time to enforce rigid dietary rules, or decide that you're only going to eat organic or nothing. If you're super tired and want a sugar hit, have it – but maybe it's worth bringing along a bar of a chocolate that you really love instead of grabbing whatever's available at the airport shop.

We like to take these on the plane:

* Nuts and seeds.

* Some chopped apples or carrots feel refreshing on a long flight.

* Bananas (these are easy to digest and also contain magnesium and tryptophan, which will help you sleep).

* Miso soup sachets – ask your flight attendant for some hot water to mix these up.

* Herbal tea bags – especially chamomile for sleep and mint for digestion.

* Homemade frittatas or muffins are great for travel (see page 236) – there's no need for cutlery and they won't leak all over your bag.

WHEN YOU ARRIVE

* Even if you drank a lot of water on the plane, travel is super dehydrating, so get plenty of liquids on arrival.

* As soon as you arrive home, or at a hotel, take a hot shower or soak in the bath with added Epsom salts (bring them with you in a ziplock bag for that first night away). To get your circulation working again, massage your scalp as you wash your hair and scrub your body with a flannel.

* After a flight, stretch gently by doing a downward dog. Or lie on a bed with your legs up against the wall; stay there for 5 to 10 minutes.

* Unpack as soon as you can, instead of living out of your suitcase while you're away. It will make you feel more grounded and settled.

* Once you've freshened up, go for a walk to get some fresh air and, if it's daytime, daylight, which will help you adjust to the new time zone.

* Stay in the new time zone as much as possible, but it's okay to get an early night or take a nap if you really need one.

EMOTIONALLY PREPARING YOURSELF FOR TRAVEL

You might think you don't have time to emotionally prepare yourself for travel – not when there's all that practical sorting to do first. But if you have time to stress out about your travel plans, you have time to prepare yourself emotionally and energetically.

* A few weeks before departure, make a to-do list to wind down your work and domestic responsibilities so there's nothing preying on your mind before you go. Do a shutdown list for the office and your home.

* Stay organised by packing well in advance. Leave your suitcase open on the floor and pack slowly for the whole week before you go. Don't do it all at the last minute and get stressed out.

* Go to bed early the night before your flight, rather than relying on sleeping on the plane. You'll feel so much better if you go to bed at a decent hour.

* Sometimes it's worth the extra money to get a flight that leaves at a regular time in the day, rather than taking the redeye.

WHEN THINGS GO WRONG
ON THE ROAD

So your plane got cancelled, or your train was delayed, or the hotel doesn't have a record of your reservation. It can be hard to deal with unexpected changes when you're travelling, especially if you're tired from the journey and in an unfamiliar environment. You can't control everything that is happening around you – no-one can – but you do have some control over how you react to it.

Try to remember that no-one set out to ruin your day. Everyone was doing the best they could, even if it doesn't feel like it to you right now. Take a deep breath, and smile, and be kind to the people you're dealing with, and hopefully they'll be kind right back.

> Nadia: *I took a little holiday to Italy and I packed my bag so carefully with everything I needed. And guess what . . . the airline lost it. I'm not usually calm in these situations, I get pissed. But that day I chose not to. When I arrived at my hotel the sun was shining. I ate a beautiful bowl of pasta. I borrowed a shirt and the hotel washed my clothes for me. And I'm very proud of myself for learning and putting into practice the things I want to be better at. Being calm, seeing things don't revolve around me, letting go of the things I can't control. And it turned out I didn't truly need one thing I'd packed. Not one!'*

NO PLACE LIKE HOME

'Love begins at home.' Mother Theresa

Your home should be your sanctuary, the place that allows you to rest, recuperate and restore yourself. Walking through the door should make you feel relaxed and calm. Does your home make you feel like that? Or do you just see the pile of ironing, or the dirty dishes stacked up by the sink?

Imagine how you'd make your house look if you had invited a special guest; candles lit, music on, fire burning, surfaces clear and dusted, cushions plumped. We always make the house nice for other people but we don't often think to do it for ourselves.

Ask yourself what you love about being a guest in someone else's home, or in a hotel. Fresh flowers? Clean sheets? A nice scented candle? Can you find the budget for one or two of these things at home?

You deserve to enjoy a house that is beautiful, with your favourite things around you. These things don't have to be expensive or fancy, you just have to love them. We like collecting little things from our travels and bringing them back to remind us of time spent with friends and family. And if you ever keep things for 'best' – whether it's plates or clothes or flower vases – get them out and use them.

Your home is your identity and it tells a story about how you want to feel in it: make that story comfortable, calm and beautiful.

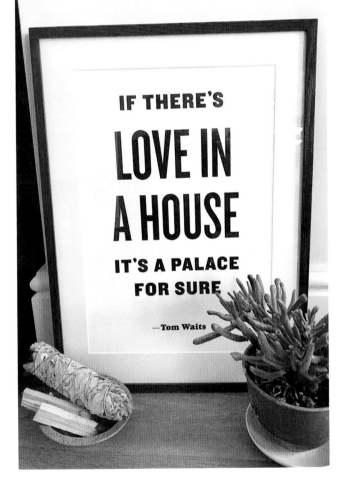

CREATING YOUR SANCTUARY

Just a few small changes to your home environment can reap huge benefits to your peace of mind.

* When you get home in the evening, change your energy from daytime to relaxation, from outside to inside. As well as taking your shoes off when you get into the house, change your clothes, too. We mean completely, even your underwear. We've got a special drawer for inside clothes: pyjamas, sweats, big cosy jumpers and soft socks.

* If you have time, take a shower or a bath when you get home. Otherwise, at least wash your hands to wash off the day. Don't bring the outside in.

* Fill your house with plants and fresh flowers, if you can. If you have a habit of killing houseplants, try a succulent, which can survive a bit of neglect.

* Crystals are beautiful and are thought to give good energy. Put an amethyst in your living room for warding off negativity, a quartz on your desk for clarity and focus, and a rose quartz in your bedroom for love and compassion.

* Even if you're renting, make your house cosy – and make it yours. Ask permission to paint the walls and hang your pictures. Buy new towels and sheets. Even if you're only there for a short time, it's still your sanctuary to come back to each day.

* Put on a vaporiser or oil burner. In the morning, use energising oils, for example, lemon, peppermint, lemongrass, basil and eucalyptus. And in the evening, swap for calming oils, such as lavender, ylang ylang, bergamot and vetiver.

* Burn sage to clear energy. This is a traditional Native American ritual which uses a stick of dry white sage (not regular kitchen sage) – you can get these online or at any health food store. If someone's been at your house crying, or there's been a drama there, burn sage and think of the negative energy leaving your space. Light the end of the sage stick and fan out the flame until it's just smoking. Either walk around the whole house with the sage stick or stand still and waft it around you. Sage is also good if you haven't been well. Make sure the windows are open and you don't go near the smoke alarms, though!

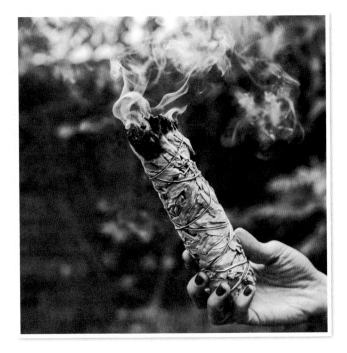

FENG SHUI FOR BEGINNERS

Growing up in Hong Kong, we were used to the feng shui man coming round to make sure everything in our home was where it should be, even down to certain walls and doors being painted the right colour. Everyone in Hong Kong does feng shui when they move house, start a business or have any other change in their life.

Feng shui may seem like a strange practice if you're new to it, but it's just about creating good energy and energy flow in your house. As with all these things, try it before you dismiss it! The worst that can happen is that your home will end up a little tidier.

Here are some of the basic principles that you can apply to your own home.

* Everything should have its place. Your home should be organised in a way that it only takes a quick tidy and wipe of countertops and tables for it to be presentable.

* Check in with your stuff and get rid of what you don't need.

* Keeping the house neat and uncluttered will help your mind feel tidy, too. If you buy something new, give something else away.

* There's usually one cupboard or drawer that you shove everything into. When you have half an hour, turn it out. Choose what to get rid of, put everything back neatly.

* Get rid of anything broken, any chipped cups or plates. In feng shui that represents cracks or troubles in your life.

* Don't let a mirror face your bed. And when asleep you shouldn't have your feet towards your door or your head towards the window.

* Go through your clothes and give away any item you don't wear any more. If you need to keep a piece of clothing but won't wear it in the next few months, put it in storage.

* Do the jobs you hate: filing, admin, etc. They take up a lot of space in your head when you know you need to do them. Ask for help if you need it.

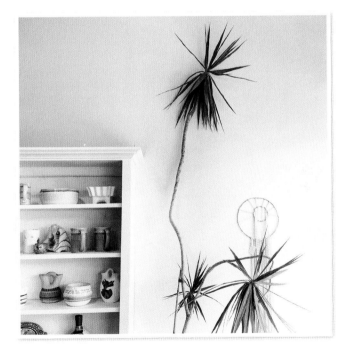

A SHORTCUT TO CALM

If you regularly light a scented candle or diffuse some essential oils when you are feeling calm and happy at home, your brain will begin to make the association between that scent and being relaxed. So at times when you're feeling frazzled you can simply light the candle or burn the oil and use the scent as a shortcut to help you quickly access that feeling of relaxation.

* When you buy aromatherapy candles, make sure they're made of natural wax and contain aromatherapy oils, not perfume.

* Use an aromatherapy diffuser and oils. There are benefits to essential oils that go beyond just the smell, as each one affects your mood and your wellbeing. There are general guidelines you can read about but it's so personal, it's really worth experimenting with what works for you. Buy all natural oils, not the ones that contain perfume.

* Fresh flowers and green plants look beautiful and smell great, too. In the winter, when it's harder to get fresh flowers, we like to scent our homes with cut eucalyptus leaves in vases.

* Add a few drops of essential oils to the water for your mop; try basil, lemon or orange. You can do the same for the water for wet-dusting your surfaces and bannisters. Add a few drops to your laundry detergent or when drying your clothes, too.

* Grow herbs if you have space: mint and basil smell lovely on a sunny windowsill.

* Bake a cake or make fresh coffee. If you're inviting people to your house, there's nothing like the smell of a cake to make people feel welcomed and looked after.

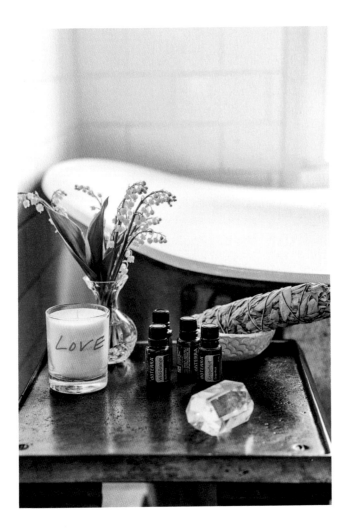

SLEEP TIGHT

'Forgive yourself each night and recommit each morning.' *Anon*

We all know what a difference it makes to wake refreshed and energised, instead of feeling sluggish and hitting the snooze button. Sleep is such a healer for your whole system; sometimes if you're struggling with a problem or an emotion you just need to sleep it off.

Yes, we're going to tell you to go to bed earlier. Not every night, but can you try to schedule in a few early nights each week? A lot of people resist going to bed earlier because they think it feels like a punishment, or that they are missing out. If that's you, we promise it's worth changing that attitude by turning bedtime into a treat. Go to bed late and you'll not only get less sleep, you'll get a less solid sleep, too.

Sleep is one of the most important elements of self-care. And that's especially true if you're going through something big, such as a loss or a break-up, depression or anxiety. Or maybe you really want to sleep but can't?

We know you'll have heard of a lot of these sleep strategies; some are very simple, but we often find people resist doing the work! This is sometimes because the solution you need may not be instant.

When you plant a seed in a pot or a garden you don't keep digging it up to see if it's started growing yet. You trust in the process and eventually the good things grow. We suggest you try some of these changes and see what happens.

Have a good night!

A GOOD NIGHT STARTS
WITH A GOOD DAY

* Get outside in daylight every day. Preferably go out in the early morning, to wake you up, and even better if it's sunny. The exposure to natural light will help regulate your internal body clock.

* Make your bed in the morning so it's an inviting place to return to when you're ready for sleep.

* Avoid caffeine after lunchtime. Try it for a week and see what happens.

WHEN YOU GET HOME

* Take a bath or shower when you come home from work, or as soon as you've eaten. Then put on your night clothes and your body will get the message that it's time to relax.

* Make sure you've finished eating at least two hours before you go to bed, or your body will still be digesting when it should be sleeping.

* No alcohol. We're not saying to give it up altogether, but alcohol disrupts your sleep and it's a good idea to give yourself several dry nights a week.

* Finish emails (especially work emails) and social media three hours before bed. If you keep remembering one more thing you need to do, just write it down instead (in pen, put the phone down!) and tackle it tomorrow.

* Turn the lights down low, wherever you are, after 9pm.

* Prepare for tomorrow – organise your bag, lay out your clothes. Make the morning easier on yourself.

* You could even prepare your breakfast the night before; we love rose chia overnight oats (see page 146).

AT BEDTIME

* Do your own turndown before bed, as if you're staying in a nice hotel. Switch on your bedside lamp, make sure your clothes are tidied away, and perhaps use a diffuser with soothing oils, such as lavender, chamomile or marjoram.

* A cool (18 degrees Celsius maximum), quiet room is best for sleep. Open a window to let the fresh air in. If your room is noisy, or if you sleep next to a snorer, try earplugs.

* The darker your room is, the better. Make sure the curtains are drawn and switch off any source of light. If it's hard to make your room pitch black, put on an eye mask.

* Put all screens in another room. The blue light from your phone or iPad interferes with the sleep-inducing hormone melatonin. If you usually use your phone to wake you up in the mornings, why not invest in an old-fashioned alarm clock instead?

WHEN YOU NEED SOME
EXTRA HELP SLEEPING

* Invest in the softest sheets you can afford and the most comfortable pyjamas (or sleep naked, whatever feels right for you!). Make going to bed a pleasure rather than a chore.

* Magnesium is known as the sleepy mineral, as it helps to relax your muscles. You can take a magnesium supplement, rub in oils or creams with added magnesium, or take a bath in magnesium-rich Epsom salts.

* Chamomile tea is a legendary sleep aid. Sip a cup before bedtime. Making the tea from whole buds, or teabags containing whole buds, will have the strongest effect.

* Make your own relaxing pillow spray by shaking 10 to 15 drops of lavender oil and/or chamomile oil in a small spray bottle of water. Or just put a drop or two of oil on your hands, rub them together, then wipe them over your pillow or sheets.

* Avoid vigorous exercise late in the evening as it gets your adrenaline going. Calming yoga with lots of deep breathing is fine.

* Try yoga nidra, which translates as 'yogic sleep'. There are many yoga nidra apps available; they will talk you through a spoken meditation which helps to give you a deep, full body and mind relaxation. It may take time to find one you like, but persevere!

* Do a big full-body squeeze and release. Lie on your back in bed, stretch your legs out, make fists with your hands, scrunch up your face and squeeze all of your muscles up tight, creating as much tension as you can in your body. Then release everything and let your body drop heavily into your bed. Do that three times.

* Try not to go to bed with any arguments outstanding, even if it means it's you who says sorry. You'll get a better night's sleep by being sorry rather than by being right.

* If you have problems with sleep, keep a sleep diary. For a week, track exercise, what you're eating, when you have caffeine, alcohol, how you feel, arguments, anxiety, that suspense-filled or violent movie or box set on your computer in bed. Then look back to see how each thing affects your sleep.

> Katia: 'If I don't get to bed by 11pm, I feel like I've been hit by a truck the next day, regardless of whether I've had a drink or not. I know what works for me is a 10.30pm bedtime. Not all the time, some late nights are totally worth it – but most of the time.'

WHEN YOU REALLY CAN'T SLEEP

There are always going to be nights when you just can't sleep. Perhaps you have trouble drifting off, or you wake in the middle of the night with your mind racing. Try not to wind yourself up by getting stressed about not sleeping – it can become a vicious circle where you keep yourself awake by fretting about being awake.

It's best not to pay too much attention to your thoughts in the small hours. This is a vulnerable time, when emotions are heightened, and you may feel gripped by fear or guilt or panic. It can help to write down your concerns in a notebook and tell yourself you'll address them tomorrow. Often these worries seem much smaller and less significant in the morning.

Try getting up and out of the bedroom for a while. Accept that you're awake right now; read a book, or make yourself a chamomile tea. This is not a time to go online (not even to google cures for insomnia). Distract yourself from panicked thoughts of 'I must sleep!' and you may find you will naturally become sleepier.

It's important to remember that long-term trouble sleeping can be a sign of something bigger, like depression. If your sleep is disturbed for longer than a few weeks, it might be time for a visit to your doctor, or a therapist.

When we can't sleep, we like to do a bedtime body scan (next page). Even if you don't fall asleep immediately afterwards, you will feel calm and relaxed.

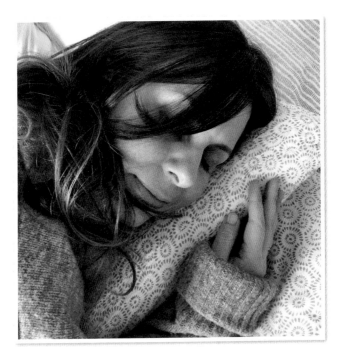

BEDTIME BODY SCAN

Lie on your back in bed with your legs comfortably apart and your arms outstretched alongside your body, palms up. If having your legs straight doesn't feel good on your lower back, place a cushion or rolled blanket under your knees. Put an eye bag or eye mask over your eyes, if you like.

Make sure you are warm enough, because as you relax you may get cold.

Take a deep breath in and release a deep sigh out through the mouth. Repeat that three times. Feel your body release into the bed.

Rest your attention on your feet and say silently to yourself, I relax my feet. My feet are relaxed.

Then go up through your whole body the same way.

I relax my legs. My legs feel heavy and relaxed.

I relax my hands. My hands are relaxed.

I relax my arms. My arms feel heavy and relaxed.

I relax my buttocks. My buttocks are relaxed.

My belly softens and relaxes. As I breathe in my belly naturally rises. As I breathe out it naturally softens.

I relax all the muscles that support my spine. All the muscles in my lower middle and upper back relax.

I relax any tension in my neck and shoulders. My neck and shoulders are free of tension and feel relaxed.

I relax my head. My head feels heavy and relaxed.

I soften my lips. I create space between my teeth. My jaw softens and relaxes.

I relax my eyes and my eyelids feel heavy. I relax my eyes.

My brain relaxes.

My whole body feels relaxed, and with each exhale I drop further into the bed.

Thank your body for all the functions it performs daily for you.

Take a deep breath in, then release a deep sigh out through the mouth.

You can repeat this as many times as you like.

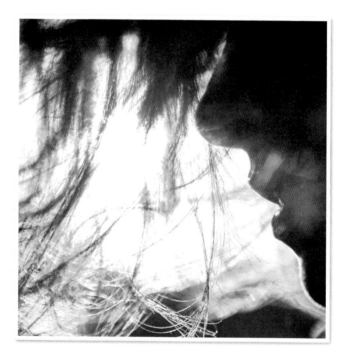

HOW TO SHINE YOUR LIGHT

* Check in with yourself. Notice how you feel. Do this every day, a few times a day if you can.

* Ask yourself, what does the sensation of lightness feel like to you?

* When do you feel you are not aligned with your light?

* Ask yourself, what would a sense of lightness and ease feel like right now in this moment?

* What could you do, right now, to shine your light brighter, for yourself and others?

* Do something today, and every day, that allows you to shine.

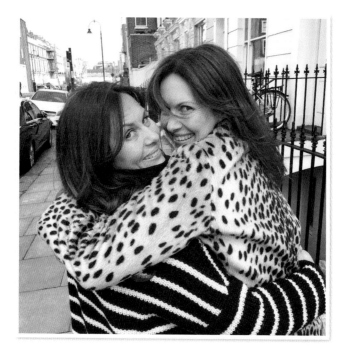

That's the end of our advice on self-care, but we hope it's just the beginning of your own journey.

Remember there is no final destination when it comes to self-care – there is no perfect self that you're going to arrive at. Think instead of a constantly evolving process towards feeling the best version of yourself, wherever you are right now.

If we can leave you with one message, it's this: LOVE, HOPE, PEACE, JOY, LIGHT are not things you have to go out and find, they're within you already. Let self-care help you find them.

ABOUT THE AUTHORS

Nadia: *Growing up I had a pretty difficult time at home and I left as soon as I could, at not quite sixteen. I was lucky enough to have a job as a model that allowed me to support myself and to travel all over the world. When I look at my friends' teenagers now, I can't believe how young I was to be out there on my own.*

Although Katia and I were fortunate to be brought up on a foundation of healthy food and exercise, I never felt that I was taught to look after myself emotionally. This, combined with being independent at such a young age, meant that I was always looking outside, to other people, for emotional stability, instead of learning to find it in myself.

When I took my first yoga class at the age of eighteen, it was like I had come home. Yoga made me feel soft and safe and held, and helped me learn a new way of being. Now I've been teaching it for over twenty years, and I'm still learning and constantly practising.

Yoga led me to meditation, which helped settle my mind. I hate how corny it sounds, like 'just practise meditation and you'll be calm', but meditation means training the mind and my mind has a tendency to be pretty volatile. So finding a practice that helped settle it was like finding a new pathway in life.

None of this was instant. It has taken a long time and many different practices, books and teachings to learn to soften my edges, to open my heart, to take care of myself and to accept myself rather than trying to fix myself.

I hope you will find this for yourself too.

@nadianarain

Katia: *Like Nadia, I left home young and did a lot of travelling. In my twenties it might have seemed as if I was having a great time exploring the world, but inside I felt insecure and uncertain. It was hard for me to feel beautiful or worthy of caring for myself; I was living with the self-destruct button pressed way down.*

My journey of self-care started with self-discovery. I was always open to alternative lifestyles, training as a reiki master, becoming a massage therapist and reading a lot of spiritual books. I began to accept that I was on a different path to the 'norm', instead of fighting it.

The big lesson I learned from all my travelling was that your unhappiness will follow you wherever you go, so you might as well be where people really love you, and face your issues and begin to deal with them.

I decided to come to London and make a life for myself with my sister and good friends by my side. My time spent travelling didn't go to waste, though; while in Hawaii I learned about raw food and juices, which led me to open my first café, Little Earth, in 2004. Now I run the Nectar Café in Triyoga, in London.

Grounding myself in London, where I live with my family, is where I'm at right now. I have learned to be comfortable in my skin and to love and accept who I am. Once this happened I found that I didn't need to run from myself anymore.

I wish the same for you.

[O] @katianarainphillips

ACKNOWLEDGEMENTS

You know we love our lists, and here's another one – all the people we'd like to thank for helping us bring this book together.

Thanks and love to Casey Phillips, for teaching us about family. And to Jonah and Huxley Phillips for being beams of love and light, and making us better humans.

Thanks to everyone at our publishers: Pippa Wright, for taking a chance on us and believing we knew what we were talking about. You have been a kind but firm editor, the perfect combination. Lizzy Gaisford for your amazing eye and all hands on deck support. Jocasta Hamilton for your big smile and constant reassurance. Najma Finlay, Jasmine Rowe and Celeste Ward-Best for all the excitement and encouragement. Melissa Four and Viki Ottewill for the perfect cover.

Abi Hartshorne, for the calm and restful design.

Brigid Moss, who gave shape to our thoughts and put our words in the right order.

Britta Jacobson, for your generosity.

Nicola Dunn, for remaining calm when we were not and always giving us a new perspective.

Carole Ingram, for your support.

Kim Sion, for capturing us as we like to be seen.

Pip Cooper and Ben Ingham, best friends and a dream team who brought beauty to our book.

Eloise Markwell-Butler and Alex Hardee, for being the perfect hosts and lending us their gorgeous home for the photographs.

Christina Wilson and Pamela Beaulieu, for your images.

Haarala Hamilton, for the food photos that made Katia cry with joy, and Emma Lahaye for working so hard and styling everything so beautifully.

Niki and Jay at Cloth House, for fabrics and friendship.

Venus Rox, for lending us the beautiful, priceless crystals.

Untitled (Flowers), for the perfect flowers.

All of the staff at the Nectar Café, and a special shout out to Josu Zabaleta for being our rainbow rolls master roller.

Michael Isted of the Herball, for help and inspiration.

Matthew Freud, thank you for showing up daily.

Lauren Phillips, without you, nothing would get done.

Gurmukh, for changing the direction of our lives forever.

Jonathan Sattin, who gave us a platform to be creative and trusted we knew what we were doing even when we weren't sure we did.

To all our teachers along the path who have taught us everything we know about self-care and caring for others.

And to the people who show up each day to classes and to the café. You allow us to wake up every morning doing what we love.

Thank you . . .

RECIPE INDEX

PICTURE CREDITS

Pages 4, 16, 43, 69, 77, 109, 110, 114, 185, 221, 225, 229 and 262 courtesy of Pip Cooper.

Pages 11, 74, 259 and 264 courtesy of Kim Sion.

Page 24 courtesy of Christina Wilson.

Pages 35, 41, 45, 47, 51, 73, 91, 93, 95, 125, 139, 143, 145, 147, 150, 160, 175, 177, 179, 181, 235, 237, 247 and 251 © Haraala Hamilton 2017.

Pages 53, 60, 81, 82, 102, 117, 133, 155, 171, 193, 195, 208 and 245 by Nadia Narain. Poster featured in photo on page 245 designed by The Bee and the Fox.

Pages 64 and 162 courtesy of Alisa Lambina.

Page 71 by Katia Narain Phillips.

Page 88 courtesy of Manizeh Reimer.

Page 107 courtesy of Pamela Beaulieu.

Page 149 from the Narain family collection.

Page 166 © Alicia Bock / Stocksy United.

Page 183 courtesy of Moni Narain.

Page 198 © Jovana Rikalo / Stocksy United.

Page 203 © Daniel Kim / Stocksy United.

Page 204 © Borislav Zhuykov / Stocksy United.

Page 212 © Kirstin McKee / Stocksy United.

Page 216 © Rolfo / Stocksy United.

Page 223 courtesy of Chris Miller.

Page 249 © Katie + Joe / Stocksy United.

Editor: Rebecca Kaplan
Design Manager: Eli Mock
Production Manager: Mike Kaserkie

Library of Congress Control Number: 2018946957

ISBN: 978-1-4197-3677-3

ABRAMS The Art of Books
abramsbooks.com

195 Broadway
New York, NY 10007
abramsbooks.com